UNBALANCED
A View from the Vestibule
Schizophrenia and Hyperattention

UNBALANCED
A View from the Vestibule
Schizophrenia and Hyperattention

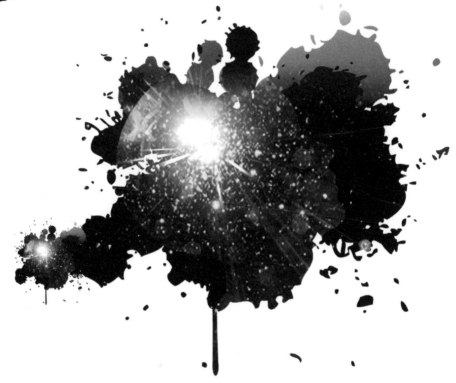

Simeon Locke

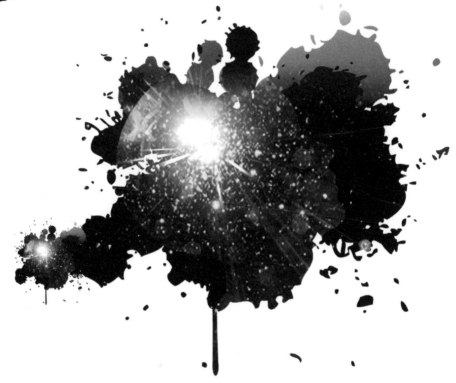

Harvard Medical School, USA

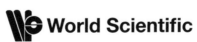

World Scientific

NEW JERSEY · LONDON · SINGAPORE · BEIJING · SHANGHAI · HONG KONG · TAIPEI · CHENNAI

Published by

World Scientific Publishing Co. Pte. Ltd.

5 Toh Tuck Link, Singapore 596224

USA office: 27 Warren Street, Suite 401-402, Hackensack, NJ 07601

UK office: 57 Shelton Street, Covent Garden, London WC2H 9HE

British Library Cataloguing-in-Publication Data
A catalogue record for this book is available from the British Library.

ISBN-13 978-981-4299-62-6
ISBN-10 981-4299-62-6

Typeset by Stallion Press
Email: enquiries@stallionpress.com

Printed in Singapore by World Scientific Printers.

CONTENTS

ACKNOWLEDGEMENTS

In some ways, what follows is a sentimental journey. Many of the ideas expressed — now brought up to date — were developed in the decade 1969 through 1979, when I was in charge of a Neurological Unit at Boston State Hospital. I had published some early ideas on the vestibular system eight years previously, but it was not until I was brought in contact with a large group of psychiatric patients that I began to think about the relation between the vestibular system and schizophrenia. In those rewarding years, we were supported by generous clinical and research grants from the National Institutes of Health and by a farsighted Hospital Superintendent, the psychiatrist Jonathan Cole, who had recently arrived from the National Institutes of Mental Health. His presence made possible the intellectual climate that allowed us to flourish. I started with nothing but an empty ward: one wing on either side of a common social area and a nursing station, six rooms — four singles, two doubles — on each wing, with space for eight patients on one side and eight offices or labs on the other. Now came the task of filling them.

First came Will Vaughn who, after graduating from college, was driving a taxi in Boston. He and I, alone in the unfurnished top floor of the medical building, set up a laboratory to do microelectrode studies on muscle. When our grant proposal elicited a site visit, we still had no furniture, no equipment and no personnel but we had enthusiasm and ideas. We had designed a stimulating–recording device that functioned through a single microelectrode, (the report of which was published subsequently in the *Proceedings of the Institute of Electrical and Electronics Engineers*) and we got our grant — much better than driving a taxi. Will went on to get a graduate degree in Psychology at Harvard and spent many years working with B.F. Skinner.

A major stroke of luck occurred in the summer of 1969. Laura Reynolds, who had recently obtained a graduate degree in psychiatric nursing, consented to accept nursing responsibility for the clinical unit. She brought an intuitive sense about people that was as important in dealing with staff as it was in understanding psychiatric patients. She put a team of bright, energetic, enthusiastic young nurses together and helped instill a non-judgmental, unretributive style of caring. We could choose our patients from anywhere in the hospital and keep them until discharge or transfer back to the ward from which they had come. It was not long before we were deluged with requests to take "unmanageable" patients because using the methods Laura had taught, our nurses could manage these unmanageables. One example will suffice. A large and somewhat threatening young women was an accomplished escape artist. Although she was kept on locked wards, they could not contain her. So, we were asked to take her in as a transfer. On arrival, Laura welcomed her and explained that because our ward was not locked she could come and go as she pleased; however, Laura also told her that in order for us not to worry, would she please let us know when she was leaving and when she planned to be back. The escapes stopped — they were no longer necessary.

Laura participated in many of the neurological and physiological ideas that were exchanged during that period, one of which culminated in a publication in the *Lancet* of a note on the relation of handedness to the onset of symptoms in postencephalitic Parkinsonism. Ultimately, she would go on to the Chestnut Lodge in Maryland, Saint Elizabeth's Hospital in Washington D.C. and then to the National Institutes of Health.

One of my major research interests during that period (which persists to this day) had to do with the vestibular system and its role in schizophrenia and in Parkinson's disease. The approach was anatomical and physiological and the cat was the experimental animal, for after all, the cat must have an extraordinarily efficient vestibular system to always land on its feet. Joyce Hilsz helped with the anatomy. Together we exposed the brain stem vestibular nuclei, injected small amounts of radioactive cocktail and subsequently, I examined the brain sections Joyce had prepared for evidence of the tracer. The physiology was done with Larry Murphy. The ampulla of the horizontal canal was exposed, brief electrical stimuli were provided and the exposed cortex and the deep nuclei were explored for response. Larry Murphy, subsequently in charge of the science department at Beaver Country Day School, moved on to being responsible for science teaching in the Weston School System and established the Advanced Biotechnology Institute at the Roxbury Latin School — a summer science program for bright youngsters who want hands-on experience.

Clearly, our studies needed several years of work and could not be completed, for conditions were changing. Jon Cole had left. Subsequent administrators were either not doctors or not interested. Strong and new social forces now appeared, to discharge as many patients as quickly as possible. "Return them to the community" was an ironic euphemism for the fact that many patients lived on the streets. State hospitals were closing. As a result, many of these ideas about the vestibular system lingered unverified and therefore unexpressed. Now, they are still largely speculative, but should not, just because of that, remain unexpressed.

Other young investigators worked with us or alone and young residents from the Boston University Neurology Program rotated through the clinical side. Steven Lipper did a study on optokinetic nystagmus in tardive dyskinesia (published in the *Archives of General Psychiatry*). Sanford Wright took a year off from his neurosurgery training to work on the anatomy of the thalamus, (several publications together with Locke and Hilsz in *The Anatomical Record* and *Brain*). Paul Brown spent a year with us before continuing his work on the tactile fields of the cat's paw, as a faculty member of the University of West Virginia.

Our interest in language led to studies with David Caplan (who went on to medical school, neurology training and is now at the Massachusetts General Hospital) and Lucia Kellar (who took a graduate degree in Psychology at Columbia) which were published in *Brain*, *Cortex* and in a monograph published by C.C. Thomas. Finally a stream of work–study students from Northeastern and Antioch colleges worked in the clinical and research sides; several have gone on to study medicine. One, Agnes Whittaker, is a pediatric psychiatrist in New York and another, Jean Matheson, who helped with the references for this enterprise (as did Laura Reynolds Cearnal) heads the Sleep Laboratory at the Beth Israel Deaconess Medical Center in Boston.

That was a fertile decade — particularly in the early years. The crops bore some fruit as the citations indicate, but a major harvest did not occur. Social conditions were wrong and the decade of the brain had not yet been declared. The effort to retrieve some of the pickings, enhanced by more recent data obtained elsewhere, accounts for the reflections that follow and the hope that the hard work of all of these people will eventuate in a lasting contribution.

PREFACE

"The advantages which have been derived from the caution with which hypothetical statements are admitted, are in no instance more obvious than in those sciences which more particularly belong to the healing art. It therefore is necessary, that some conciliatory explanation should be offered for the present publication: in which, it is acknowledged, that mere conjecture takes the place of experiment; and, that analogy is the substitute for anatomical examination, the only sure foundation for pathological knowledge.

When, however, the nature of the subject and the circumstances under which it has been here taken up, are considered, it is hoped that the offering of the following pages to the attention of the medical public will not be severely censured. The disease, respecting which the present inquiry is made, is of a nature highly afflictive. Notwithstanding which, it has not yet obtained a place in the classification of nosologists; some have regarded its characteristic symptoms as distinct and different diseases, and others have given its name to diseases differing essentially from it; whilst the unhappy sufferer has considered it as an evil, from the domination of which he has no prospect of escape." I ... "therefore considered it to be a duty to submit [these] opinions to the examination of others even in their present state of immaturity and imperfection."[1]

So wrote James Parkinson in 1817 in *An Essay on the Shaking Palsy* (Fig. 1), which was later to become an eponymous disorder as suggested by Charcot. I quote him at length because I too am going to write about Parkinson's disease. I am also going to write at much greater length about schizophrenia, which is the major interest of this undertaking. If you parse the quote carefully, you may well decide it applies equally to schizophrenia.

Why discuss Parkinson's disease and schizophrenia in the same breath? Because, I will argue, they may be but two instances of a disorder of the same system. In one case, Parkinson's disease is a deficit of function. In the second case, schizophrenia is an excess of activity to account for the positive symptoms and perhaps a deficit of activity in relation to the negative symptoms.

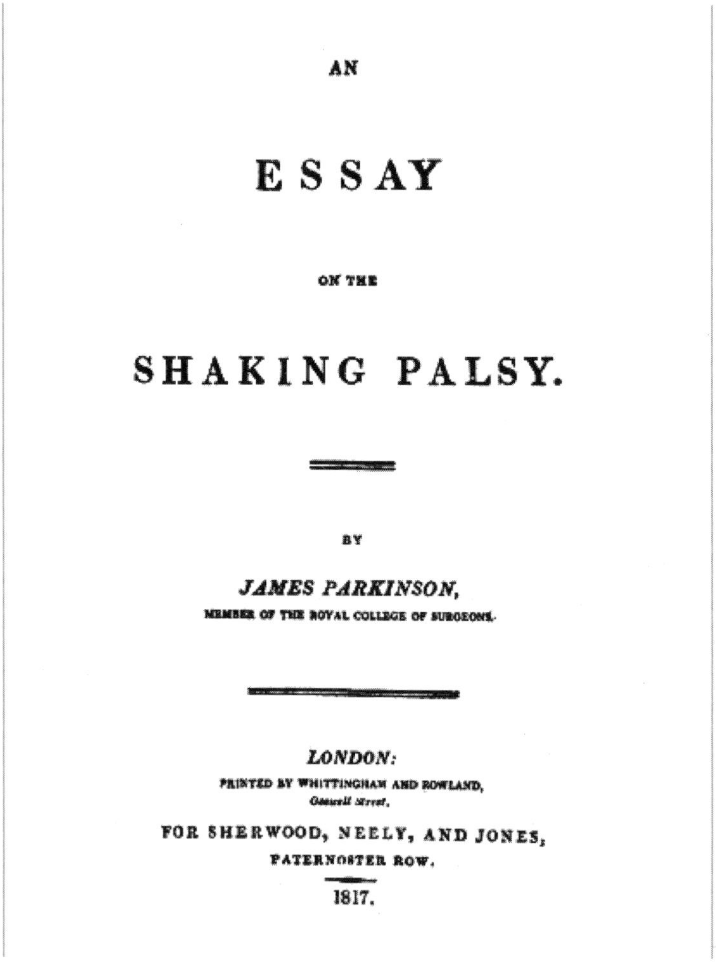

AN

ESSAY

ON THE

SHAKING PALSY.

⸻

BY

JAMES PARKINSON,
MEMBER OF THE ROYAL COLLEGE OF SURGEONS.

⸻

LONDON:
PRINTED BY WHITTINGHAM AND ROWLAND,
Goswell Street,
FOR SHERWOOD, NEELY, AND JONES,
PATERNOSTER ROW.
1817.

Fig. 1. Title page of James Parkinson's 1817 essay on the disease that has come to bear his name.

The activity is generated by the arousal system, that was originally designated the mesencephalic (or more accurately pontomesencephalic or brain stem) ascending reticular activating system, which is now understood to include structures rostral to the mesencephalon.[2] This nonspecific system receives input from collaterals of many of the specific systems including somatic and visceral sensation, vision, audition and most importantly to our argument, vestibular. In addition, reticular neurons send projections to spinal cord from ventromedial medulla and caudal pons,[3] a point of presumed importance in disorders characterized by heightened muscle tone: the rigidity of Parkinsonism, the so-called "waxy flexibility" of catatonia, and the loss of muscle atonia during REM sleep behavior disorder.

The ascending system can be conceived as having two parts: an arousal system that wakes the brain and a clock that wakes the arousal system. The clock, an early evolutionary acquisition present in plants as well as in animals, is primarily based in the suprachiasmatic nucleus, is free-running but can be set. The most powerful agent is light, particularly blue light, which not only entrains the clock but quite promptly increases alertness and attention.[4] The effect of light has been demonstrated in Seasonal Affective Disorder and abnormal circadian rhythms have been claimed for schizophrenia.[5] The entrainment pathway (Fig. 2) is from non-image forming melanopsin containing retinal ganglion cells that, by the retinohypothalamic tract, project to the suprachiasmatic nucleus and adjacent areas. These, in turn, project to the subparaventricular zone of hypothalamus, which, by way of the median forebrain bundle, sends fibers to the inter-mediolateral horn cells of the upper dorsal segments of the spinal cord. Preganglionic fibers from these cells terminate in the superior cervical ganglion and the postganglionic fibers project to pineal gland to control production of melatonin, which can entrain the suprachiasmatic nucleus.

The reticular system is a very old system. In evolutionary progression, as judged from comparative anatomy, it antedated the development of specific sensory pathways. It is a diffuse network of nuclei and fibers on both

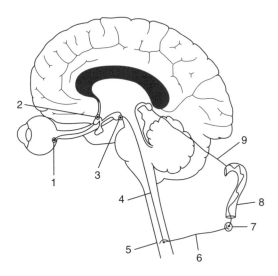

Fig. 2. Neural pathways of the clock (schematic): 1: Non-image forming, melanopsin containing retinal ganglion cell; 2: Suprachiasmatic nucleus; 3: Paraventricular nucleus of hypothalamus; 4: Medial forebrain bundle; 5: Intermediolateral horn cell uppper dorsal spinal cord; 6: Preganglionic sympathetic fibre; 7: Superior cervical ganglion; 8: Carotid artery; 9: Postganglionic sympathetic fiber; 10: Melatonin producing pineal.

the input and output sides of the nervous system. The later developing lemniscal system conveys modality-specific impulses in well-defined tracts, paralleled on the output side by the late-developed corticospinal tract. Each lemniscus conveys a single modality by way of the thalamus (except in the case of olfaction — a very old modality) and then projects from the thalamus to specific cortical areas. The cortex appears as an areal mosaic of the primary sensations — vision, audition and somatic sensation. Along their courses, each fillet gives off collaterals that lose their modality markers before contributing to the brain stem reticular formation. It is this general sensory input to the reticular activating system that constitutes the initial input to the arousal system then distributed by its component nuclei widely to cerebral cortex. A dorsal path projects to the thalamic nonspecific nuclei (particularly the intralaminar nuclei), which are interspersed among the specific thalamic nuclei of the lemniscal systems. A ventral pathway passes by way of the hypothalamus to the basal forebrain to terminate in cells in the substantia innominata, the medial septum and the diagonal band, which in turn project widely to the cerebral cortex. Among the inputs to the reticular formation are some that do not come to consciousness. Prominent among these is the vestibular input. Vestibular input differs from most sensory input in that we are only aware of it when it goes awry. It functions tonically (it is always discharging), but it reaches conscious awareness only when the discharge of the two sides is unequal. It serves as a null indicator with no conscious awareness on the part of its possessor of the level at which it is set. The result of firing rapidly or firing slowly is the same for the sensory (or specific) aspect as long as the two sides are in balance. But the nonspecific aspect, as seen by the arousal system, may be very different in each instance. If set high, the subject may be hyperalert, excessively aroused, and extremely vigilant. Seeing too much and hearing too much may express itself as the positive symptoms of schizophrenia — hallucinations and paranoia. If set low, the specific component may function poorly, leading to problems with balance and posture. The nonspecific component may be deficient, causing decreased attention, lack of initiative, and because the medial and the descending vestibular nuclei normally produce inhibition of reflex tone in limbs by way of the reticulospinal path, the lack of spontaneous neural activity may account for the rigidity of Parkinson's disease or the negative symptoms of schizophrenia: apathy, blunted affect, emotional withdrawal and most strikingly, rigidity of catatonia.

Compare the two: the overactive vestibular system of the paranoid hallucinating schizophrenic with the underactive vestibular system of the rigid, bradykinetic Parkinsonian:

Schizophrenia	Parkinson's disease
Loose Association	Rigid Thinking
Flight of Ideas	Obsessive Ideation
Disorganized Behavior	Compulsive Repetition
DOPA Blocker Therapy	DOPA Replacement Therapy

Eye movements which are ultimately connected to the vestibular system, are abnormal in both conditions. Sleep patterns are abnormal in both and sleep is an expression of function of the reticular system. Hallucinations occur in both — whether from too much DOPA (therapeutic or endogenous) or from the dreamlike state of an inactive reticular activating system.

So, that is the hypothesis. It is at a level between the molecular or genetic on is one hand and the clinical on the other. It de-emphasizes without ignoring the role of transmitters, not because transmitters are unimportant, but because ultimately it is not transmitters that produce behavior. Transmitters implement activity by modules or networks of neurons, which are responsible for the correlate of behavior and it is by behavior that we judge the presence of schizophrenia or Parkinson's disease. The hypothesis is an effort to give a biological base to a psychiatric disorder and to understand the psychological aspects of a very different biological disorder. It may not be right but it should be testable. As James Parkinson said almost two centuries ago: "To delay... publication did not, indeed appear to be warrantable. ...The task of ascertaining [the] nature and the cause by anatomical investigation, did not seem likely to be taken up by those who, from their abilities and opportunities, were most likely to accomplish it. That these friends to humanity and medical science, who have already unveiled to us many of the morbid processes by which health and life is abridged, might be excited to extend their researches to this malady, was much desired; and it was hoped, that this might be procured by the publication of these remarks."[1]

Chapter 1

DISEASE

Disease, we were told in medical school, comes in three categories: (1) poor make; (2) bad luck; (3) worn out. This classification may be as good as any for a comprehensive definition of disease is hard to come by. We think we know what we mean as long as we do not look too carefully. This is particularly true in the case of psychiatric disease where objective signs are often lacking. Certainly, disease is a deviation from normal but not all deviation is disease. The notion of normal is ambiguous because it has moral as well as statistical overtones. Is normal good and abnormal bad? Can one extreme of the normal distribution curve be good and the other extreme be bad? Take intelligence for instance. Or is the mean the normal and all deviations bad? The dictionary is of no help: To be "free of disorder" or "not abnormal" is to offer only tautologies. "Although medicine has come a long way from the day when a ten-volume work could be written upon nosology — as witness the classic of Sauvage — it still lacks philosophical precision when it comes to the definition of a 'disease'… In many fields of medicine, it must be frankly admitted that our conception of this or that 'disease' is a purely fictional one; an artifact, even though of value."[6]

If the standard is not statistical, not population, can it be the individual? Can deviation from a former condition become criterion? Only if the former condition was good or was normal, so here we are again. Dementia is abnormal because it is a decline from a former mental capability, but how about amentia or other congenital anomalies (I avoid the word "abnormality"), or even such common things as weight loss? Loss of weight from 300 pounds to 150 pounds for an average-sized individual is good, a return to normal, but loss of weight from 120 pounds to 75 pounds for an average-sized individual is bad, is abnormal; and both causes — bulimia and anorexia nervosa — are bad, are abnormal.

Not only is the notion of "normal" statistical and moral, but it is also social. Society imposes standards that may be arbitrary and may become criteria. Thin is pretty, fat is not, although it is more acceptable now than it was

1

50 years ago in America. These social criteria, so important for psychiatric diagnosis, vary from generation to generation, from culture to culture, and from language to language. Homosexuality was a disease until recently. American enthusiasm, which might be viewed elsewhere as mania, contrasts with British phlegm, which some might consider blunted affect. Mania and blunted affect are criteria of psychiatric diagnoses. Not very long ago, the prevalence of schizophrenia in the United States was twice of that in Great Britain,[7] which really means the diagnosis of schizophrenia in the United States was twice as high, a statement about diagnosis, not about schizophrenia. This cultural or social aspect of the norm is what allows Thomas Szasz, and perhaps R.D. Laing, to argue that psychiatric patients are not ill, just different.[8] Laing in "The Divided Self", claims that society is sick and that "schizophrenia is a rational response to a mad society".[9] Psychiatric diagnoses based on social (actually societal) criteria can be and have been used for political purposes. Dissidents may be hospitalized as psychotic,[10] or even killed.[11]

A "scientific" approach to disease might demand objective evidence but the presence of evidence may reflect the state of the art as well as the mode of thinking. For example, gastric ulcer, once thought to be of emotional etiology, is now realized to be bacterial. Some diseases are structural — that is due to disordered anatomy — and some are functional — the disorder is of physiology. The two may go together but need not. Functional disorder may occur in the absence of observable and anatomical change; structural abnormality may occur without disruption of function. As techniques develop, more functional (in the sense of psychological) disorders became organic. Others, such as cardiac arrhythmias or epilepsy, may have known structural correlates. The challenge of the schizophrenias is to delineate the access routes to the underlying organic pathology.

One recent attempt approaches the task from the aspect of homeostasis. Homeostasis is defined as a "dynamic physiological cognitive and affective steady state that integrates...sensory afferents" with "cognitive and affective control processes resulting in dynamic stability."[12] Decision making, a function of the brain, in this formulation changes the homeostatic state, and in this formulation, "decision making dysfunctions in individuals with psychiatric disorders." This is not really objective and like so much of science, it simply restates a truism. You do not have to undertake a study to discover that psychiatric patients, particularly the hospitalized ones, often make poor decisions and bad choices: the fact that they are hospitalized shows that.

How about genetics? A recent report[13] relates that a gene for brain development plays a role in schizophrenia. Nerve cell migrations, a usual occurrence, might be disturbed if the gene (labeled DISC1) is altered or lacking and one of its binding partners transmits nerve signals into cellular responses necessary for memory. "Memory and cognition are both disturbed in schizophrenia.[13] But genes and their expression (such as brain wiring) differ in individuals, so "normal" still remains a social definition without objective "scientific" criteria. Human genetic variation was termed by the journal, *Science*, as the "breakthrough of the year" for 2007. The article started with the phrase, "Researchers are finding out how truly different we are from one another", and ends with the phrase, "Such structural and genetic variety is truly the spice of our individuality."[14] These differences are "normal".

An early attempt at objective criteria for bacterial disease was Koch's Postulates. Koch, who won the Nobel Prize in 1905, postulated four things: (1) Microorganisms must be found in abundance in all organisms suffering from the disease but not in healthy organisms. (2) Microorganisms must be isolated from a diseased organism and grown in pure culture. (3) The cultured microorganism should cause the disease when introduced into a healthy organism. (4) The microorganism must be re-isolated from the inoculated diseased host and identified as being identical to the original specific causative agent. Objective perhaps, but notice how "healthy" rather than "normal" becomes the ambiguous term as Koch discovered when he found that "healthy"carriers of typhoid and cholera exist.

One way of classifying disease is whether the process is intrinsic or extrinsic. Is something like Koch's microorganisms added to the body or is something taken away? Bacterial pneumonia, AIDS, toxic states (whether internally created or consumed from outside), are all extrinsic. Something has been added. Alzheimer's disease, tremor and athetosis, stroke and paralysis are situations where something has been subtracted. The distinction is between positive and negative, but this should not be confused with positive and negative symptoms or positive and negative mechanisms or processes. Symptoms and signs of schizophrenia (symptoms are what the patient experiences; signs are what the doctor sees or hears or palpates) are classified as positive or negative. Positive symptoms — hallucinations or delusions, for example — do not mean something has been added to the body (unless you believe in spirits). Ironically, the deluded schizophrenic who believes in control by radiowaves or cosmic forces believes something has been added. The negative symptoms of apathy, flat affect or catatonia do not mean that something has been taken away. The process may be negative and release a positive result — movement disorder from nervous tissue destruction, for example, or may be positive and cause a negative result — loss of consciousness, (negative) from a seizure, a positive discharge of nerve cells.

The disorders that we will explore in the following sections are all intrinsic. Nothing has been added. Whatever comes out was in the body to start, was present but obscured in the normal. This means that the study of normal mechanics may be revealing, that substraction from normal mechanics may release some unanticipated positive symptoms as the result of a negative process. It may mean that some abnormal phenomenon may be released in the normal under certain circumstances, dreams for instance, emphasizing once again the social criteria that determine what is normal.

The social aspect of disease is put in relief by Sontag who writes of illness as a metaphor. Not only is illness determined by social attitudes, but social attitudes are also determined by illness. Cancer, she writes in 1978 "is felt to be obscene". It is "abominable, disgusting, offensive to the senses". In contrast, "cardiac disease implies a weakness, trouble, failure that is mechanical; there is no scandal."[15] And so, for psychiatric disease, which has many parallels with tuberculosis, a disease as dreaded in the past as cancer is today, "in both diseases there is confinement. Sufferers are put in a 'sanitorium', the common word for a clinic for tuberculars and the most common euphemism for an insane asylum. Once put away, the patient enters a special world with special rules. Like TB, insanity is a kind of exile. The metaphor of the psychic voyage is an extension of the romantic idea of travel that was associated with tuberculosis. The patient has to be taken out of his or her daily world. It is not an accident that the most common metaphor for an extreme psychological experience viewed positively — whether it is produced by drugs or by becoming psychotic — is a trip."[15]

The distinction, indeed separation, of physical and mental illness is yet one more demonstration of the persistence of Cartesian dualism in our thinking. Despite its problems, the success of psychopharmacology in the treatment of psychological disease makes it evident that psychological illness is organic, that disease of the mind and disease of the brain are but two manifestations of a single process. How the two relate (really translate) from one to the other — brain to mind — is the crucial question. This is simply another expression of a fundamental unresolved (and perhaps unresolvable) philosophical problem — the conversion of the physical to the psychophysical, the neuronal to the perceptual, the somatic to the psychic. It is interesting that the converse, once very much in fashion, never presented the same philosophical problem. Psychosomatic illness, the conversion of a mind function to a body function, was generally accepted although "illness" was still not defined.

The effort to define psychiatric illness objectively resulted in the publication by The American Psychiatric Association of the *Diagnostic and Statistical*

Manual of Mental Disorders, familiarly known as the DSM-IV. The current fourth edition offers a checklist to make diagnoses of schizophrenia more objective. The psychiatrist is told what is needed for the classification to be tenable. Subjective factors are allegedly controlled, but subjective factors really remain. If flattening of affect is an objective criterion of schizophrenia, the decision of whether an affect is flat is a subjective decision of the psychiatrist. Or, for example, disorganized speech; talk to any adolescent (although some might argue that adolescence is a self-limited form of schizophrenia). Further complications (never mind what you think of a checklist approach) are that schizophrenia may not be a single disease but a group of diseases. Bleuler, who coined the term in 1908, spoke of the "schizophrenias", suggesting a number of different entities.

Before Bleuler, the situation was chaotic. Thirty different systems of classification existed up until the time of Morel in the mid-nineteenth century. One, that of Guisling in Belgium, included about one hundred different states. A unitary hypothesis appeared before Hughlings Jackson, but his emphasis on positive and negative manifestations of neurological lesions had great influence on subsequent thinking and was rather different from the mosaic approach of Wernicke, Kleist and Leonhard, just as Jackson's ideas about aphasia were quite different from Wernicke's. In 1863, Kahlbaum published his monograph on "The Grouping of Psychological Illnesses and the Classification of Mental Disorders". He differentiated two large groups. One, designated as a limited disturbance of mind, was remitting and the symptoms remained stable over time. This group included mania and depression. The second group presented progressive symptoms and ended in dementia. Catatonia was considered a subgroup of this larger classification. Kahlbaum's effort to separate disorders with a favorable prognosis from those that presaged dementia, forecast the seminal classification of Kraepelin who argued for a somatic cause of psychiatric disease but realized that lack of knowledge about causation made classification and prediction difficult. Nonetheless, in the fifth edition of his textbook he relates disease to causation, symptoms, course and outcome. In that text, he published a chapter on dementia praecox, and in the next edition (Fig. 3), he integrated Kahlbaum's catatonia, included hebephrenia, which had been described by Hecker in 1871, and distinguished dementia praecox from manic depressive psychosis.[16] This had a long lasting effect. Until recently, catatonia has been considered a manifestation of schizophrenia. The problem relates in part to the fact that there is no consistent definition of catatonia.[17] For many, it is defined by the motor phenomenon; most often this is perseveration of posture, less often a hyperactive manic state. For Kahlbaum, the alteration of mood was primary

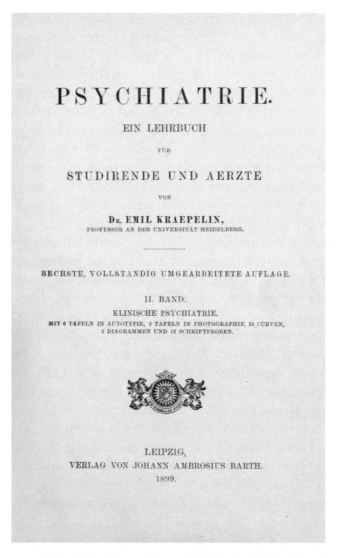

Fig. 3. Title page of the sixth edition of Kraepelin's *Textbook of Psychiatry for Students and Physicians*. In this edition he integrated Kahlbaum's catatonia.

and the motor symptoms a manifestation. These motor symptoms may appear in a number of disorders other than schizophrenia in which 5% of the cases first diagnosed are catatonic. But catatonia is also found in affective psychosis as well as in toxi-metabolic encephalopathies, drug intoxications, frontal lobe e.g., third ventricle lesions, disorders of the basal ganglia, degenerative disease and limbic lesions including encephalitis. DSM-IV recognizes the association with disorders other than schizophrenia.[18] The wide array of etiologies is mimicked by the wide array of manifestations, both negative and positive.

Motor signs of posturing, rigidity, and waxy flexibility are accompanied by mutism and staring, or agitation, combativeness, and impulsive behavior. Repetitious movements, grimacing, echolalia and echopraxia occur just as they do in Parkinson's disease. Non-ictal discharges have been postulated as responsible for tremor and rigidity in Parkinsonism in a circuit involving thalamus and globus pallidus — a self-perpetuating tonic oscillation. Benzodiazepines, used to treat seizures, are also effective in treating catatonia; anticonvulsants are used in the treatment of bipolar disorder, the major cause of catatonia.[19]

Kraepelin's desire to find a biological cause for psychiatric disease went unfulfilled despite participation by skilled morphologists such as Alzheimer and Nissl. The distinction he proposed between dementia praecox and manic depressive disease has been challenged, in part because criteria such as catatonia are found to be widespread.[20] Kraepelin knew this. In 1920, he wrote of "the difficulties which prevent us from distinguishing reliably between manic-depressive insanity and dementia praecox. No experienced psychiatrist will deny there is an alarmingly large number of cases in which it seems impossible, in spite of the most careful observation, to make a firm diagnosis...it is becoming increasingly clear that we cannot distinguish satisfactorily between these two illnesses and this brings home the suspicion that our formulation of the problem may be incorrect" (quoted in Ref. 21).

Kraepelin's assumption that dementia praecox irreversibly ended in dementia and that patients with manic depressive disorder recovered led to Bleuler's introduction of the term "schizophrenia", for he had experience with schizophrenics who recovered. Despite the inability to demonstrate anatomic abnormality in brain, Kraepelin continued to consider dementia praecox a degenerative disorder, for he said, "Degeneration certainly plays a part in the development of dementia praecox."[22] The conclusion is still held.[23] "The persistence of aspects of the degeneration theory, despite much contrary evidence, is an example of how one can be imprisoned by an archaic way of thinking,"[22] which brings us back to Susan Sontag, never mind "the body of evidence that symptoms apparently characteristic of psychosis are common in the general population, i.e., in people who are never formally considered either by themselves or others to suffer from an illness."[21] Once again, we confront the issue of disease, or normality, and of the lack of objective evidence.

Perhaps the best one can do is accept the fact that psychiatric diagnosis reflects a social attitude, realize that the patient — the so-called sufferer — is really suffering and, as a compassionate physician, try to ameliorate the suffering. Often this is hard to do, for the medication we think makes the schizophrenic better is often rejected by the patient who does not like the symptoms but does not like the treatment even more. It may be that the symptoms have a reason — an argument that might be offered by an analytic psychiatrist. They certainly have a cause. That cause is in the brain (ultimately, of course, in the genes) and should be discoverable. The job for the moment is to continue the search.

Chapter 2

AROUSAL

If the postulate that an abnormality in the activating arousal system has any merit, based in part on clinical observation but also on the knowledge that arousal is associated with increased forebrain serotonin,[24] and if an important contribution to the activating system is the vestibular component, then an analysis of each of these systems is necessary.

For clarity, the discussion of arousal should be divided into two parts, one dealing with the ascending activating system, the second with the pacer or circadian (about 24 hours — *circa diem*) clock. The arousal system determines the rest — activity cycle of the organism. The clock does considerably more. It regulates such things as body temperature, hormone production and feeding.[25] One concern not usually verbalized is that much of the information has been derived from studies on nocturnal or crepuscular animals and then has been applied to humans, in whom light is an important factor for setting the clock. An internal clock is a very old evolutionary achievement. It is present in plants, fungi, and unicellular organisms. It has a widespread distribution in higher creatures for in a given individual it is present in many tissues and organs, which, while under the control of the "concert master", the suprachiasmatic nucleus of the brain which determines that the individual tissue pacemakers function in concert — the local pacemakers can be entrained separately. So, for example, the liver's clock can be entrained by feedings.[26] Rhythmicity, independent of brain, has been identified in heart, liver, kidney and lung. It has even been demonstrated *in vitro* where the oscillations are no longer in phase.[24] The major regulator is made up of neurons that behave as individual circadian pacemakers and function together, one with the other. The individual cell process (physiologic not anatomic) is autonomous which, by interaction with other cells, becomes coherent. The coherent process is free running; it occurs in the explanted suprachiasmatic nucleus maintained *in vitro*. In the animal, the nucleus sits just above the optic chiasm to the side of the third ventricle. It has a small-celled dorsomedial part called "the shell" and a larger-celled ventrolateral division spoken of as "the core". Each nucleus communicates with its fellow on the other side. The roughly 24-hour period of the free running oscillation can be entrained. Photic and non-photic stimuli serve. Social cues, feeding time, hormones and locomotor activity are among non-photic entrainers. Melatonin, secreted by the pineal gland, is one such agent. However, light is far and away the major factor. Melanopsin-containing retinal ganglion cells,[27] which are intrinsically photosensitive, form the retinohypothalamic tract which projects to the suprachiasmatic nucleus and send collaterals to the intergeniculate leaflet, a homologue of the pre-geniculate nucleus of man. Most input, which is bilateral, is to the ventrolateral division of the suprachiasmatic nucleus, which also receives rich input from the intergeniculate leaflet,[28] but the dorsomedial division receives some as well, as do other hypothalamic areas. From the suprachiasmatic nucleus, projections are sent to the homolateral subparaventricular zone and from there in the basal forebrain bundle to the intermediolateral horn cell of the upper dorsal spinal cord. Preganglionic fibers project to the superior cervical ganglion from which postganglionic fibers are distributed with blood vessels to the pineal. There, the elaboration of melatonin responds to the light–dark cycle and is fed back to the suprachiasmatic nucleus to facilitate entrainment.[29,30] The intergeniculate leaflet, a distinct subdivision of the lateral geniculate complex,[31] which receives retinohypothalamic tract collaterals, is also part of the light entraining pathway. By way of the geniculohypothalamic tract, it projects predominantly to the core of the suprachiasmatic nucleus. It contributes to visuomotor circuits: oculomotor, trochlear, anterior pretectal, Edinger–Westphal, superior colliculus, interstitial nucleus of the medial longitudinal fasciculus, periaqueductal gray and others. Locus coeruleus and medial ventricular nucleus which contribute to sleep and eye movement regulation and which project to the intergeniculate leaflet, do not receive reciprocal projections.[32] The intergeniculate leaflet may not exist in humans.[33]

The effect of light is immediate, long-lasting and greater for green and blue than for other wavelengths. It serves to alert the brain, to enhance cognitive activity and allegedly functions in frontal and parietal cortex as well as in the brain stem region of the locus coeruleus.[34,35] The effect is by way of a non-image forming visual system which responds to shorter wavelengths than does the visual system.[36] Exposure to light during biological night suppresses melatonin production and produces activity of the parieto-occipital cortex in proportion to the duration of the light exposure.[37]

Entities other than light influence behavior arousal. Stress, hunger, and emotion are known to contribute. Orexin-producing neurons of the posterior hypothalamus may play a role as they are known to innervate arousal-promoting regions of the brain. They project to the spinal cord and diffusely in the brain by way of the thalamocortical and basilocortical systems, and to the monoaminergic nuclei of the brain stem. Input to the orexin-producing cells comes from many hypothalamic regions: claustrum, lateral septum and allocortex.[38]

The activating system first came to prominence with a 1949 publication of the relation between reticular brain stem stimulation and cortical arousal.[39] Often discussed as if it were a system in itself, two points, though obvious, should be made. First, it is an afferent system that connects the brain to the environment. Second, the afferent input, which is not modality marked, is by way of collaterals from the modality marked lemniscal systems.[40] The brain stem components, the nuclei, can be classified according to transmitters. This classification allows extension of the reticular activating system beyond the confines of brain stem and now includes hypothalamus and basal forebrain (Fig. 4). The major transmitters are monoaminergic, cholinergic, histaminergic, and glutaminergic. Dopaminergic neurons are prominent in the substantia nigra, ventral tegmental area, and ventral periaqueductal gray.[41] They project to the striatum, basal forebrain, nucleus accumbens, septum, amygdala and frontal cortex and are important in behavior arousal. The major noradrenergic projections are from the locus coeruleus which projects widely to the cerebral cortex, the brain stem as well as to the spinal cord and is associated with cortical arousal.[42] Serotonergic neurons of the dorsal and median raphé nuclei are concerned with photic entrainment. Two groups of cholinergic neurons project to the forebrain. One, the lateral dorsal tegmental and the pedunculopontine tegmental, projects to the intralaminar thalamic nuclei, to the basal forebrain and to the lateral hypothalamus. The second, the nucleus

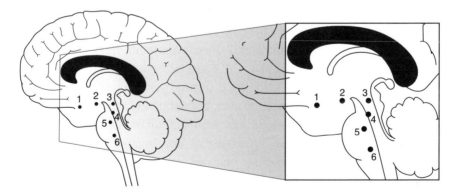

Fig. 4. The ascending reticular activation system. Schematic view nuclear components: 1: Ventrololateral preoptic nucleus (VLPO); 2: Tuberomammillary nucleus (TMN); 3: Laterodorsal tegmental nucleus (LDT); 4: Peripedunculotegmental nucleus (PPT); 5: Raphe nucleus; 6: Locus ceruleus (LC). Cholinergic; 3, 4, aminergic; 5, 6, histaminergic; 2, GABAergic; 1.

basalis of Meynert, the nucleus of the diagonal band, the septum and the substantia innominata, projects widely to the cortex. The first travels in a dorsal thalamic pathway, the second in a ventral extrathalamic pathway. Histamine-containing neurons are found in the tuberomamillary nuclei and adjacent posterior hypothalamus. They project widely to the cortex and are associated with wakefulness. Glutamate is the predominant excitatory transmitter in the brain involved in reticular, thalamic and cortical projections. It is the major transmitter to the perifornical orexin containing neurons, which are a prime component of the activating system and are also influenced by cholinergic and GABAergic basal forebrain terminals.[43]

Obviously the activating system is but one part of a two-state system, the other face of which is sleep. This is why sleep is examined in schizophrenia, for it provides an access route to the arousal system which may be disturbed in schizophrenia. As von Economo recognized long before the discovery of the reticular activating system, sleep and its converse are generated in the hypothalamus. From his study of cases of encephalitis lethargica, he concluded, "The inflammation in cases associated with insomnia is localized anteriorly in the lateral wall of the third ventricle, near the corpus striatum, while it is localized in cases showing disturbances of the ocular muscles with sopor in the posterior wall of the third ventricle near the nuclei of the oculomotorius in the cap of the interbrain."[44] As sleep reflects the state of wakefulness, it is not of concern to our argument so it will be treated only briefly. It consists of two major categories, rapid eye movement (REM), and non-rapid eye movement (NREM) sleep, the latter of which is divided into four electrographic stages correlated with the depth of sleep. NREM sleep is largely regulated by the anterior hypothalamus, particularly by the ventrolateral preoptic nucleus, which sends gamma-aminobutyric acid-mediated inhibitory impulses to the wake-producing nuclei, including the histaminic tuberomammillary nuclei and the cholinergic pedunculopontine as well as the lateral dorsal tegmental nuclei. A subpopulation of these nuclei (peripeduncular, PPD and laterodorsal tegmental, LTD) is active during REM sleep and is inhibited during wakefulness by the aminergic arousal neurons. The medial preoptic area, the subparaventricular zone, and the dorsal medial hypothalamic nucleus relay suprachiasmatic nucleus output to the sleep-promoting nuclei in the ventrolateral and median preoptic nuclei.[45] During REM Sleep, the aminergic neurons are switched off. A region of the mesopontine tegmentum contains GABAergic REM — on sublaterodorsal tegmental nuclear neurons and ventrolateral periaqueductal GABAergic REM — off neurons. From the REM on area, projections to basal forebrain regulate electrographic desynchronization during REM sleep. A second projection to the ventromedial medulla and the spinal cord is associated with muscle atonia.[46]

On this background, I would like to once again propose that a fundamental defect in schizophrenia relates to the function of the reticular activating system. Presumably in most cases, it is overactive for although it is not possible to draw direct conclusions from the nature of the symptoms (positive or negative) as to the nature of the reticular activity (overactive or deficient respectively), it is likely that an overactive reticular system can result in either positive or negative symptoms; an underactive reticular system will produce only negative symptoms. That both negative and positive symptoms may exist in a given patient at the same time precludes postulating two separate mechanisms.

If the reticular activating system is overactive in this disorder, there are two possibilities to consider that account for the overactivity. One is that the afferent input is excessive, that the gain is set too high prior to arrival of the projected information in the reticular activating system. Were that so, the specific and nonspecific aspects of the input would reflect it. The image-forming capacity of the visual system would be as affected as the non-image forming capacity. Similarly with the auditory system. Lights would appear too bright, sounds too loud. Now it is true that the schizophrenic suffers distortions of reality and may report an excess of stimulation by the visual or auditory systems but this does not require the interpretation of increased input at the first links in the chain — receptors and initial afferent neurons. While this might account for the heightened perception, the amplification may take place beyond the initial stage.

Among the sensory systems that project to the reticular activating system, the vestibular system has a special place. Its input is no different from that of other sensory systems. The difference occurs at the first stages of the system. Most sensory systems project a direct representation of what they transduce or experience to higher levels. A brighter light or a louder sound results in a bigger specific output. Not so with the vestibular system, for it is a balanced system as well as a tonic one. It is always active but only comes to conscious perception when it is unbalanced. Motion or position are only perceived when the position of the cristae or otolith of one side is not offset by the position of the cristae or otolith of the other side. It is the difference of discharge level on the two sides that accounts for the perception of movement or position, not the level of discharge itself. The difference of level is appreciated by way of the specific system; the absolute level is recognized by the nonspecific system where it may generate further activity. When the vestibular input is high, the reticular activating system activation may be high but the primary abnormality is in the vestibular, not the activating system. The increase of input would not be known as it would were it to occur in the

visual or the auditory systems, which simultaneously convey the same information to specific and nonspecific symptoms. The input to activating and
balance systems is different; one, an addition, the other, a subtraction or algebraic summation. There seems to be no way to test this directly in humans.
The observation that eye movements are abnormal in schizophrenia or even
of a difference of response to vestibular stimulation does not absolve the reticular activating system from being the primary site. Sensory systems receive
feedback; the vestibular system receives efferents. Fibers project from the
medial and the lateral reticular formations, raphé nuclei, pontine reticular formation, subcoeruleus area and many other regions in the reticular
formation.[47] Thus the possibility of an abnormality early in vestibular input
must remain speculative.

The likelihood of the disorder originating in the reticular activating
system should be explored as well. A number of factors favor such a construction. For a start, the reticular fibers of the reticular formation, in contrast
to the well-myelinated aggregated fillets of the lemniscal systems,
are thin, unmyelinated, and with rare exception (the median forebrain bundle and the posterior longitudinal fasciculus of Schütz — and even those
are loosely aggregated) form a meshwork, a reticulum. Many of the fibers
have varicosities which contain vesicles and are thought to secrete non-
synaptic neuromediators. Many cells of the reticular formation contain
neuropeptides including cells in the periaqueductal gray, the locus coeruleus
and the parabrachial nucleus. Neuropeptides — and there may be more than
one in a given cell — coexist with a classical transmitter such as noradrena-
line, serotonin, acetylcholine, gamma-aminobutyric acid. The action of
neuropeptides on behavior is one of long duration following slow onset. The
modifying effect amplifies or attenuates the influence of classical transmitters.
Thought to stand between focal and fast synaptic transmission by myelinated
nerve bundles and slow, prolonged and diffuse endocrine communication,
these modulators are released from non-synaptic regions of an axon into
non-synaptic regions of a dendrite. This long-duration non-synaptic communication among thin non-myelinated fibers does not preclude specificity of
response and allows economical use of the neuropil. Non-synaptic exocytoses
and receptor complexes on non-synaptic surfaces of the neuron have been
documented. In addition, there are gonadal steroid-receptive neurons in
the forebrain and the brain stem, including the medial preoptic nucleus, the
ventromedial hypothalamic nucleus, the periaqueductal gray, and the
parabrachial nucleus.

The general notion then, is that the presence of hormonal and neu-
ropeptide receptors — an endocrine and paracrine system of neuronal

communication respectively — implies a different method of communication from other parts of the brain. The onset of schizophrenia in adolescence and the presence of gonadal steroid receptor neurons in the brain stem reticular formation is of interest, but of greater interest is the multitude of neuropeptides (at least 16) whose action on brain stem neurons is of slow onset, long-duration and most importantly, it determines the level by amplifying or depressing the effect of the classical transmitter.[48] If the gain is set too high in the nonspecific reticular activating system, perceptual distortions by the specific afferent systems will occur, presumably at the highest stages where the systems coalesce. So one looks to cerebral and probably cortical levels beyond the primary projection fields as the place for hallucinations, perceptual distortions and paranoia to occur.

This explanation runs into difficulties when dealing with catatonia, its stereotypy — echolalia, echopraxia, persistence of posture and rigidity — so reminiscent of postencephalitic Parkinsonism. Perhaps some insight can be obtained by looking more closely at that disorder and its most characteristic manifestation, the oculogyric crisis which may be initiated with vertigo.[49] The crisis can be conceived as a perseveration of eye posture, a rigidity of movement which, like catatonic rigidity, is reversible. The reversibility, the episodic character, whatever else it means, indicates a neural discharge, whether excitatory or inhibitory. The discharge itself, of course, is excitatory. An inhibitory discharge indicates excitation of the inhibitory fiber. The inhibition is of the next neuron in the chain. If by analogy with postencephalitic Parkinsonism in which there is hypolabyrinthine sensitivity,[49] catatonia is considered a negative symptom reflecting a negative process with release of phenomena represented at a lower level, then one place to look would be at the inner segment of the pallidum, for it is known from the toxic form of Parkinson's disease associated particularly with carbon monoxide or in experimental animals with carbon disulfide,[50] of the vulnerability of the pallidum. The striatum, which is alleged to be involved in schizophrenia, receives dopaminergic input from the substantia nigra, the affection of which (pars compacta) is related to the symptoms of Parkinson's disease. Striatal efferents project to the pallidum and then back to cortex via the thalamus to constitute an important motor circuit. In addition, from the ventral pallidum there are projections to the arousal system, to the periaqueductal gray, the lateral hypothalamic area, and the mesencephalic locomotor region.[48] This subcortical motor system also receives input from the brain stem including the dorsomedial reticular formation, the vestibular nuclei, the interstitial nuclei and more. It is concerned with, among other things, eye and neck movements and thus is a logical place to consider as involved in the oculogyric crisis. The ultimate genesis of the oculogyric crisis must be in the brain stem for that is where the nuclei and tracts coordinating eye movements are found. A proposed loop might be the dopaminergic nuclei of the reticular formation to the substantia nigra, striatum, pallidum, and back to the reticular formation, with the episodic crisis representing an interruption of this loop. Where the episode is generated need not be in the loop, which can be viewed as a closed-loop with open-loop input, but in light of the hypothalamic predilection of encephalitis lethargica, the occurrence of oculogyric crises in some of the acute cases, and the finding of acute hypothalamic inflammation, the hypothalamus might warrant consideration. An inhibitory discharge, perhaps from the GABAergic ventrolateral preoptic nucleus of the hypothalamus, could initiate the episode but the discharge would need to be restricted to the dopaminergic nuclei. In this view, catatonia can be conceived as a circumscribed episode of Parkinsonism.

Chapter 3

PARKINSON'S DISEASE

For convenience, Parkinson's disease has been grouped in four varieties: (1) The idiopathic form described by James Parkinson called "paralysis agitans". (2) The presumed viral form which followed encephalitis lethargica, and thus called "postencephalitic Parkinsonism". (3) A toxic variety caused by agents such as manganese, carbon monoxide or most frequently, phenothiazines or butyrophenones. (4) A vascular variety associated with small vessel disease the so-called "arteriosclerotic Parkinsonism". Each form differs from the others and has specific clinical and pathological features. From each of these, I will select the aspects of interest for our discussion and omit those which do not pertain, so this will not be a complete clinical description of any one of the varieties. Tremor, the agitans of paralysis agitans and the hallmark of the disorder, for example, will not appear. The symptoms that cross-boundaries of the four categories are problems of equilibrium, bradykinesia or slowness of movement, rigidity to passive manipulation of body parts, and difficulty initiating action. Tremor or other movement disorder may be present, abnormality of eye and eyelid movement may be evident and compulsive behavior often appears. Flexed posture is a cardinal sign of the idiopathic form, less common but present in the others; indeed, dystonia in extension may occur in the postencephalitic or toxic varieties.

To start with the last variety in order to discard it, arteriosclerotic Parkinsonism results from multiple lacunar infarcts, particularly in the globus pallidus, a border zone between the small vessels on the convex of the hemisphere that dip into cerebral white matter and the small vessels at the base that extend up. The region where these two territories meet appears particularly vulnerable to toxic lesions as well. Indeed, the small vessel lacunae simply indicate the vulnerability to oxygen-lack caused by reduced blood flow as the pallidal lesions in carbon monoxide poisoning indicate the vulnerability to oxygen-lack caused by reduced blood oxygen-carrying capacity. The outstanding clinical feature of arteriosclerotic Parkinsonism is bradykinesia and the rigidity of *Gegenhalten*, a counter-pull rather different from the rigidity of paralysis agitans. The incidence of arteriosclerotic Parkinsonism is declining,

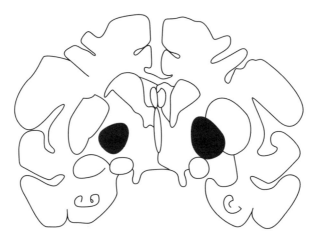

Fig. 5. Monkey brain showing effect of experimental carbon disulfide exposure. Globus pallidus (black) is necrotic. Similar necrosis was present in the substantia nigra. The damage is sharply circumscribed; adjacent structures are spared. Affected animals showed signs of Parkinsonism, including flexed posture of trunk and limbs, rigidity and tremor.

perhaps as a result of improved treatment of hypertension. This form of Parkinsonism does not figure in our discussion so it will be put aside.

The toxic form of the disease has some interest largely because of the behavioral aspects. Once again, the pallidum is the site of major affection. Not only does carbon monoxide preferentially affect the pallidum, but so does manganese with predilection for the inner segment, while hypoparathyroidism may cause bilateral pallidal calcification with symptoms of Parkinsonism (Fig. 5). Pesticides have been implicated. Clearly, a focal cause for a behavioral disorder cannot be postulated in the presence of a diffuse toxin, but it is interesting that behavioral disturbance, psychosis and hallucinations have been reported as "manganese madness" or as "locura manganica".[51] My own experience is more concordant with the obsessive compulsive behavior of other forms of Parkinsonism. In the mid 1950s, I did a clerkship at the Salpetriere on what once had been Charcot's service. There, I saw a patient with manganese intoxication. As he lay in bed, he would touch his nose with his right forefinger every so often, perhaps every minute or two, and then return his arm to his side. As we spoke, I gently rested my hand on his right forearm. Shortly, he touched his nose with his left forefinger. "Why do you touch your nose?" I asked. He could not explain, but in response to my next question, he said he could refrain. I asked him not to touch his nose and he agreed. As he talked, he gestured increasingly in ever expanding arcs until with one emphatic gesture, he touched his nose. Then his gestures quieted down. As his disease got better, his compulsion disappeared. Manganese, a much more common toxic agent in the past, has again made an appearance with striking changes in the globus pallidus, substantia nigra, and substantia innominata, on imaging studies in users of methcathinone, attributed to the potassium permanganate used in its manufacture.[52] The relationship of the pallidum to the vestibular system was stressed by classical neurologists.[53]

The most common toxic agent nowadays is the so-called major tranquilizers. These dopamine blockers manifest their neurological effect most evidently in movement disorders which do not mimic the tremor of paralysis agitans. Buccolingual dyskinesias are common, oculogyric crises may occur, choreoathetosis may be unilateral or bilateral and an extended body posture is not unusual. Dyskinetic response to phenothiazines occurs in four ways: (1) An idiosyncratic response in which a single therapeutic dose, usually the first, produces a dramatic and often long-lasting dyskinesia — buccolingual or ocular. (2) A dose-related response in which signs appear as the dose is increased and disappear as the dose is decreased. (3) A dose-related response in which signs appear as the dose is increased and do not disappear as the dose is decreased. (4) Tardive dyskinesia in which the signs do not appear until late in treatment and then persist or worsen as the drug is withdrawn. These four response patterns emphasize the differences in our nervous systems and may point, once again, to the notion that schizophrenia is not a single disease. Methylphenyltetrahydropyridine (MPTP) is selectively toxic to the dopamine-bearing neurons of the pars compacta of the substantia nigra and is used to create animal models of Parkinson's disease.

Postencephalitic Parkinsonism is a sequel of encephalitis lethargica described initially by von Economo. He encountered it first in 1916, although epidemics of a similar disorder had been reported as early as the 1500s.[54] Clinically, he reported three presentations, the most common of which was characterized by severe somnolence. Sleep from which the patient could be roused might last for weeks and was accompanied by prominent eye signs of nuclear palsy. A second form was the converse — a hyperkinetic, hypermanic insomnia perhaps accompanied by chorea or myoclonus. The least common presentation was a rigid bradykinetic form of Parkinsonism, even in the acute phase. Most commonly however, the signs of Parkinsonism appeared later, sometimes years after recovery from the acute phase in which headaches were often prominent. Temporally, the disease occurred during the period of influenza pandemics, so a viral etiology had been postulated, although no virus has ever been demonstrated. There is however, an interesting report of influenza virus antigen in the postencephalitic Parkinson brain in six specimens studied by immunofluorescence.[55] A persistent chronic infection has been postulated on the basis of diffuse astrocytic reaction in archival cases,[56] which offers one explanation for the delayed onset of Parkinsonism. A recent study of an alleged cohort of 20 new patients suggests an autoimmune basis.[57] Neuropathologic study in the acute phase demonstrated nerve cell destruction, perivascular and meningeal infiltrate in the mesencephalic periaqueductal gray and posterior hypothalamus in the somnolent form in which oculomotor nuclei might be included. Late stages showed fibrillary changes in oculomotor nuclei and substantia nigra. Anterior hypothalamus and basal ganglia were affected in the insomnia form. Degeneration of the substantia nigra was found in late cases with depletion of cells in the locus coeruleus, midbrain, raphé nuclei and pontine tegmentum, nucleus pontis centralis caudalis, and nucleus raphé interpositus. Neurofibrillary tangles appeared in pedunculopontine nucleus. Neuronal loss and gliosis occurred in the hippocampus, entorhinal cortex, amygdaloid complex, thalamus, hypothalamus and subthalamus. Periaqueductal gray, supratrochlear nucleus, dorsal tegmental nucleus, locus coeruleus, and lateral dorsal tegmental nucleus were all affected. Of six recently examined cases, the vestibular nuclei were spared in all,[58] suggesting that signs attributable to the vestibular system arise from abnormality in the amplification of vestibular input rather than in the vestibular nuclei themselves (a question considered but not resolved in the previous chapter on arousal), a conclusion concordant with the affection of many nuclei of the arousal system. However, van Bogaert cites Schaller and Oliver as having demonstrated lesions in the region of the vestibular nuclei, lesions in the nuclei themselves, and lesions in the nuclei that connect with the vestibular nuclei by the medial longitudinal fasciculus.[53]

Sleep disorder continued into the postencephalitic phase with such things as reversal of the sleep–wake cycle, daytime somnolence, sleepwalking, and episodic stupor. Autonomic abnormalities including salivation, bladder dysfunction, and appetite changes were reported. Obesity occurred, a point of some interest, as leptin, a hormone that functions in the hypothalamus to reduce appetite, apparently functions in the substantia nigra as well for the substantia nigra pars compacta, which is affected in postencephalitic Parkinsonism, has an abundance of leptin receptors.[59] Respiratory abnormalities included tics such as coughing, sniffing or occasional barking. Movement disorder was common, but the characteristic three-per-second resting tremor of paralysis agitans was not. Often asymmetrical, dystonia, athetosis or chorea were grafted on a usually flexed but occasionally on a hyperextended trunk. Rigidity with decreased associated movement accompanied the abnormal postures, even though the posture, for example an athetoid hand, would suggest hypotonia. Akinesia with little spontaneous postural adjustment was common and movements, when they occurred, were slow. Compulsive movements were common, the most frequent of which were the oculogyric crises. Usually preceded by a sense of impending something — the patient was never able to describe the sensation but knew that something was coming — the eyes would turn conjugately to one side or the other (for a given patient, usually the same side), and then up. Diagnosing this as a compulsion could be demonstrated by demanding the patient look elsewhere. With sufficient exhortation, the fixed posture would be relinquished only to be resumed when the exhortation was discontinued. Moaning or occasional shouting would accompany the episode as might palilalia, also a compulsion, which would persist only as long as the crisis, though persistent echolalia or palilalia may appear without crises in the postencephalitic or idiopathic variety of the disorder. With the crises, which usually lasted about 30 minutes but could be prolonged, the patient often had an obsessive thought that went round and round like a tune that cannot be shaken off. Patients are often reluctant to talk about these ruminations but my impression is that for a given patient, it is usually the same thought in each episode. For example, one (now elderly) woman would recall an occasion when her boyfriend brought her home after a date. Her thought during each crisis was, "I think I said, but I know I didn't say 'F me Bill'." Compulsive palilalia was demonstrated by one woman who was moaning during a crisis:

"Rosemary, how do you feel?" I asked.
"Terrible doctor, terrible doctor," she replied.
"Why do you talk double?" I inquired.
"I don't know, I don't know," she said.
"SAY I DON'T KNOW." I demanded.
"I don't know," she said softly.
"Very good," I complimented her.
"Thank you doctor, thank you doctor," she replied.

Schilder,[60] quoting Stengel, says that during the oculogyric crisis, changes in the caloric irritability of the vestibular apparatus are very common.

Compulsive repetition, not true palilalia, also occurs, perhaps with other compulsions. As often as Mabel (a patient) would put her tongue back in her mouth, it would compulsively be drawn out again. On rounds we would ask, "How are you today Mabel?" To which she would reply, "Sittin' around takin' a little nourishment". Repeat the question and we get the same reply. This would happen six or seven times in rapid succession until she would terminate the episode with the remark, "Ah, come on". If compulsive behavior truly reflects obsessive thought, rigidity of thought contrasts sharply with the loose associations ascribed to the schizophrenic.

Despite the prominence of sleep disorder in postencephalitic Parkinsonism, little dynamic information is available. This is partially because the clinical distinction between postencephalitic Parkinsonism and paralysis agitans is not always made in the absence of a definite history of encephalitis. In part, this is because polysomnography did not become generally available clinically until the 1970s. A discussion of the polysomnographic abnormalities of sleep and dreaming will be combined with that for paralysis agitans. Similarly, with eye movement abnormality, prominent in both the idiopathic and the postencephalitic form of the disorder; except for the oculogyric crisis, little distinction is found between the eye movement abnormalities in the two forms of the disease, although blepharospasm is suggestive of the postencephalitic variety.

The outstanding aspects of paralysis agitans are the flexed posture, bradykinesia, rigidity with loss of associated movements, tremor at rest and difficulty with equilibrium as seen in festination. On pathologic grounds, the disorder has been divided into six stages.[61] The disease is a synucleinopathy in which a misfolded protein, alpha-synuclien, aggregates in the soma and processes of certain nerve cells as Lewy bodies and Lewy neurites. These inclusions appear long before clinical symptoms of Parkinson's disease become evident. Except for olfactory neurons (and sense of smell is often impaired in paralysis agitans), sensory nerves are spared. Motor neurons are vulnerable with a predilection for cells with long, thin, poorly myelinated axons in contrast to cells with thick, heavily myelinated axons which are not involved. It is suggested that the large fibered cells are protected because they require less energy; they are more stable because of interaction with oligodendroglia and less susceptible to pathological sprouting. An alternative way of viewing the vulnerability however, relates to use. We know, from Sister Kenny's experience with poliomyelitis, that use predisposes the destruction of the motor neuron by the poliomyelitis virus. Presumably, this reflects a membrane alteration associated with use. We have suggested[62] there may be a relation between use and onset of symptoms in postencephalitic Parkinsonism similar to that seen in focal dystonia of writer's cramp, violinist's cramp and old-fashioned telegrapher's cramp. In his "Essay on the Shaking Palsy," Parkinson comments on the onset of symptoms in a limb subject to considerable exertion (his case 1). Thinly myelinated fibers are customarily the processes of small cells. Small cells have a lower threshold than large cells.[63–65] In the synucleinopathies, the affected cells tend to be always active, as the early-onset of abnormality in the dorsal motor vagal (an autonomic) nucleus and the olfactory nerves suggest. Normally, alpha-synuclien binds to synaptic vesicles; when the disorder occurs, alpha-synuclien loses its ability to bind to the vesicle, changes its formation, aggregates and appears as Lewy neurites or bodies. What causes the change (perhaps it is a change in synaptic vesicle membrane) is not evident, but the speculative relation to use cannot be resisted. This speculation recalls the spectre of excitotoxicity in which cell death is a consequence of activity. Two points to keep in mind are: (1) The presence of Lewy bodies may signal the presence of abnormality, but may or may not be the cause of abnormality. (2) The lack of Lewy body does not signal the lack of abnormality; the abnormal cell may not form Lewy bodies for another reason. In Stage 1 of the disorder, the dorsal motor vagal nerve cells that connect with the also involved vasoactive intestinal polypeptide neurons of the enteric plexus (remember James Parkinson noted: "The bowels…had been all along torpid") and the olfactory complex are affected. In Stage 2, the lower raphé nuclei, the gigantocellular reticular nucleus and the coeruleus–subcoeruleus complex are involved. Normally these nuclei, among other functions, regulate the sensitivity and excitability levels of spinal motor neurons "possibly placing them in a heightened state of preparedness for action."[61] In Stage 3, the process moves from pons to midbrain and forebrain involving the substantia nigra, the tegmental peripeduncular nuclei, the oral raphé nuclei, magnocellular nuclei of basal forebrain and the tuberomammalary nucleus of hypothalamus. In the transition to Stage 4, which affects the temporal mesocortex, the earliest clinical signs may appear to become fully expressed by Stages 5 and 6 when sensory association and prefrontal cortical fields show changes (Fig. 6).

A consequence of the synucleinopathy of paralysis agitans is the impairment of function of the dopaminergic pathways. The pathway of particular

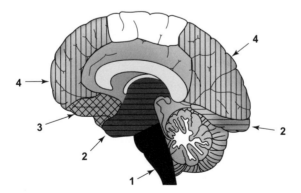

Fig. 6. Stages in the ascending synucleinopathy of idiopathic Parkinson's disease beginning in brain stem and ascending to high level neocortex. The disorder becomes apparent clinically in Stage 4 when the process affects substantia nigra and amygdala. Numbers show the progression of the process in time.

interest is from the substantia nigra pars compacta to the striatum and then to the globus pallidus, for there is reason to implicate the pallidum in the characteristic flexed posture.[50,66] The argument is that spinal section produces a posture of flexion. For extension, the vestibular nuclei must participate as shown by the decerebrate rigidity released by the section above the vestibular nuclei but below the red nucleus. A proposed pathway is from vestibular nuclei to thalamus in the mesencephalic tegmentum between the medial and lateral lemnisci.[67] A thalamic waystation in the magnocellular medial geniculate nucleus projects to the pallidum. The deficient vestibular participation caused by pallidal lesions contributes to the disorder of equilibrium and of postural recovery seen in both paralysis agitans and postencephalitic Parkinsonism. This does not mean a deficit of labyrinthine function as postural defensive reactions persist even when apparent labyrinthine function is lost.[68] This may represent compensation by proprioceptive mechanisms or compensation by central vestibular structures as shown by Bechterew over a century ago.[68] The vestibular deficit may occur anywhere along the input circuit. Monkeys with bilateral pallidal lesions have problems with balance. That the problem is a central one in postencephalitic Parkinsonism is shown by the failure of postural adjustment in patients with normal proprioceptive and labyrinthine functions when tested on a tilt table.[67]

If the hypothesis of the vestibular system's role in Parkinson's disease and schizophrenia is correct, it should be manifested as abnormalities in eye movements secondary to the intimate connections between the vestibular nuclei and the medial longitudinal bundle. Response to rotation, caloric stimulation, vestibulo-ocular reflex, and optokinetic nystagmus could assess this. Alterations in limb tone might be anticipated as a manifestation of the descending reticulospinal path abnormality secondary to the contribution of the vestibular nucleus. An alteration of arousal manifest by change in sleep architecture as a result of changes of input to the reticular activating system from the tonically active vestibular system as should be demonstrable.

Eye signs are legion in Parkinsonism. Without distinguishing the idiopathic from the postencephalitic form, J. Lawton Smith[69] lists 25 eye signs, the most important of which are paresis of upward or downward gaze or of convergence or of accommodation. Oculogyric crises are noted. Wilson's sign is that conjugate lateral movement is possible only when the eyes are blinked. Saccadic eye movements, says Smith, are simply ocular manifestations of cogwheeling, a term used to describe the rigidity of limb, and the disturbance of saccadic eye movement is thought to be a manifestation of bradykinesia.[70] Vertical supranuclear gaze palsy and eyelid apraxia is associated with pathological changes including neurofibrillary tangles and threads in brain stem.[58]

Reduced blink, blepharospasm, retracted eyelids and ptosis occur spontaneously or the first two can be induced by tapping the glabella. Finally, vertical optokinetic nystagmus dissociation occurs, in which upward or downward optokinetic nystagmus may be impaired while the contrary motion is preserved, and there may be impairment of the vestibulo-ocular reflex. The intimate connections between the vestibular pathways (more than just the medial longitudinal fasciculus), eye movements and the location of the pathology, particularly in the postencephalitic form, helps understand these phenomena. Of particular interest is that the same pattern of eye tracking dysfunction is found in Parkinson's disease (type unspecified) and schizophrenia (type unspecified).[71]

"Sleep becomes much disturbed", Parkinson writes. The onset of sleep disorder correlates with the appearance of Lewy bodies in the brain stem even before evident clinical signs. REM sleep behavior disorder may antedate the appearance of signs of paralysis agitans of which it is a harbinger. In contrast, the marker for sleep disorder in postencephalitic Parkinsonism is the neuropathology in the hypothalamus. In paralysis agitans, the monoaminergic projections are affected, particularly the dopaminergic neurons of the substantia nigra, along with the serotoninergic neurons of the dorsal raphé and noradrenergic neurons of the locus ceruleus. Cholinergic neurons of the pedunculopontine nucleus are reduced and they are thought to partake in REM sleep, where the fragmentation of sleep occurs with increased latency, frequent wakings, reduced slow wave sleep and reduced REM. The reduction of Stage 3 and Stage 4 sleep occurs in untreated patients so it is a not a manifestation of therapy. Although tremor is reduced or suppressed during slow-wave sleep, it occurs in Stages 1 and 2, with awakenings and before or after the transition to REM. Sleep benefit is noted by about one-third of the paralysis agitans patients who feel better in the morning than later in the day without any evident change in sleep pattern. Daytime sleepiness has been ascribed to the disorder,[72] but the effects of therapy are hard to eliminate.

The effects of medicine also intrude in the form of dreams, nightmares, hallucinations, and what has been termed "drug-induced psychosis" to emphasize perhaps, that Parkinsonism lacking dopamine is the obverse of schizophrenia. Daytime hallucinations may coincide with daytime sleepiness, a REM intrusion producing dream imagery perhaps followed by post-REM delusions.[73] This dissociated REM sleep is considered a breakdown of state determining boundaries of sleep. Patients may appear awake or asleep but there is twitching, vocalization and reports of dreams. Electrographically, there is a mixture of elements of wakefulness, REM sleep and NREM sleep.[74] Behavior disorder may occur in REM or non-REM (NREM) sleep, but it is

the REM sleep behavior disorder that is specifically associated with the synucleinopathies and is often a predecessor of overt Parkinson's disease. REM
sleep behavior disorder implies a dissociation of the components of REM
sleep, for the motor behavior indicates a loss of atonia. In fact, independent
pathways for the atonia and the EEG desynchronization of REM sleep have
been demonstrated.[46] The two components of REM sleep behavior disorder,
a vigorous dream accompanied by vigorous motor activity, are present in the
patient with Parkinson's disease despite the rigidity and bradykinesia of
the disorder. About a third of Parkinson's disease patients are reported to
have REM sleep behavior disorder,[75] and the fact that it often antedates overt
symptoms and L-DOPA treatment removes therapy from consideration as a
causative factor. Rather, it is attributed to an abnormality in the dopaminergic pathways — a unifying factor in all the synucleinopathies.[76,77]

The major point to take away from this survey is the evidence for involvement of the vestibular system in Parkinson's disease. The flexed posture, the
deficit of postural readjustment, the imbalance, the rigidity, the multiple eye
signs, all point to a deficit of direct (or specific) involvement of vestibular
input. The flexed posture, deficit of postural readjustment and imbalance, is
vestibular deficit by way of the pallidum, which is a focal point "since the
other ganglia appeared to act through it".[66] The rigidity is by way of medial
and descending vestibular nuclei, which activate a reticulospinal inhibitory
path by way of the lateral vestibular nucleus, which ordinarily projects by way
of the lateral vestibulospinal tract monosynaptically to the extensor alpha
motor neurons of spinal cord to activate them.[78] The multiple eye signs point
to vestibular contribution to the medial longitudinal bundle, including input
from the medial vestibular nucleus during REM sleep.

The indirect or nonspecific vestibular input to and projections of the
pontomesencephalic–hypothalamic system accounts for the ponto-geniculo-
occipital waves (PGO) or "the stuff that dreams are made of",[79] which indicates the disorder of sleep including nocturnal insomnia, daytime sleepiness,
REM intrusions with hallucinations and post-REM delusions. In passing,
note should be made that hallucinations of Parkinson's disease are usually
visual in contrast to schizophrenia where the hallucinations are often auditory. Three speculations that follow are: (1) The decrease of vestibular input
(along with the decrease of other sensory input) contributes to the decreased
output of the dopaminergic system which is deficient (if only as shown by the
therapeutic response to L-DOPA in the non-arteriolosclerotic forms of the
disease), in Parkinson's disease. (2) The rigidity of thought that occurs in
Parkinson's disease even before the onset of dementia (perhaps as a signal of
oncoming dementia) is a reflection of (or reflected in) the rigidity of muscles.

It has always seemed to me that the inability to shift, to be flexible, presaged the oncoming dementia of any etiology. A useful demonstration (quick, easy and not bulky) is the Weigl–Goldstein–Scheerer blocks: Four plastic squares, four triangles and four circles, one of each colored yellow, one red, one blue and one green are given to the patient with the instruction to put those together which belong together. Once grouped, the patient is asked why it was done that way. The expected answer is the abstraction, that blocks were grouped by shape (form) or by color. [The explanation, "I put all the squares together," etc. or "all red ones together" is considered more concrete and not as high level]. Now comes the important step. "Can you group them another way?" the patient is asked. Inability signals dementia may be on its way. Sometimes a patient who has responded to the original instruction with the question, "You mean by form or by color?" once having grouped the blocks, is locked in and cannot shift. Do rigidity of thought and rigidity of muscle belong together? Is the perseveration of posture and the Gegenhalten often seen in non-Parkinsonian dementia a coincidence? (3) Labyrinthine destruction produces circling behavior in animals. Obsessive thinking is recurrent. "The thought goes round and round in my head," we say. A metaphor or an insight?

Chapter 4

SCHIZOPHRENIA

In 1893, the German psychiatrist Emil Kraepelin grouped three types of adolescent psychiatric disorders — hebephrenia and its disorganized thinking, catatonia and its immobility and paranoia with its delusions — under a single rubric. He called it "dementia praecox" (although it is suggested[80] dementia praecox was introduced by Morel in 1860). Dementia because he thought it to be a disorder of the brain and praecox to contrast it with senile or late-life dementia. At this point, Alzheimer had not yet published his report of a case of presenile dementia. Because of brain deterioration, Kraepelin predicted these patients would never get better. The brain deterioration was inexorable. So years later when Eugen Bleuler was confronted with patients who got better, he understood it to mean the process was reversible and the brain was not permanently damaged. He renamed the disorder "schizophrenia" and referred to it in the plural entitling his 1911 text, *Dementia Praecox or the Group of Schizophrenias* (Fig. 7). The split mind of schizophrenia was a "splitting of the psychic functions", an inability to distinguish reality from fantasy,[81] and was construed as an impairment of perception of reality. Bleuler also expanded the classification to include a fourth type, called "simple schizophrenia". This basic classification persists, though the terms have changed somewhat and it has been expanded. Hebephrenia is now termed "disorganized" and "simple" is called "undifferentiated". A fifth subtype has been added: "residual" — the patient who has been treated successfully but has some symptoms left over.

Phases of the disorder are now recognized. The acute phase may last hours to years, the phase of stabilization where symptoms decline and the patient begins to resume normal function may last six months or more and the stable phase is characterized by lack of or few residual symptoms. The lack of objective criteria in a diagnosis hardly needs repetition as the utility of a checklist of the sort offered by DSM-IV is arguable[7] and the participation of cultural, social and linguistic standards in diagnosis is evident. This was driven home to me when I was assigned oversight of a unit of chronic patients after our Neurological Unit at Boston State Hospital had closed. Units were

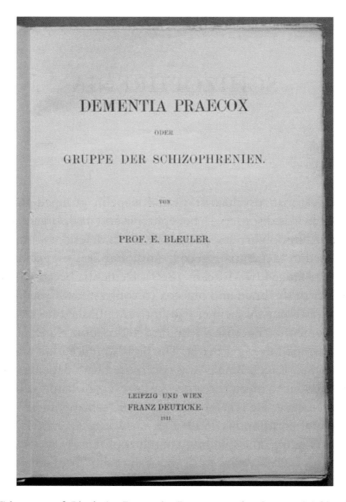

Fig. 7. Title page of Bleuler's *Dementia Praecox or the Group of Schizophrenias.* The classification proposed in this 1911 text presists to the present with only minor revision.

responsible for catchment areas in the community and mine was Roxbury, a poor, predominantly black neighborhood. I came on the ward one day and, as always, the television sets were on full blast, radios were blaring, patients were shouting, the input level was intolerable. Thinking about the question of information overload in schizophrenia, I gently suggested to the head nurse — a black woman — that it might be therapeutic to reduce the noise level. She said, "That's the way you live, that's not the way we live". I had forgotten that even in a single city, there are cultural and linguistic differences that are important in diagnosis and treatment. A footnote to all of this — particularly to the phases of the disease and to the effects of neuroleptic therapy — is to keep in mind that my experience is entirely with chronic patients who had been treated for some time even if they were not on medication at the moment. Persistence of phenothiazines in the body for months after cessation of therapy is well documented.

Two-thirds of the cases of schizophrenia appear between the ages of 17 and 25, earlier in boys than in girls. Adolescence is turned on by an as yet undiscovered putative clock. The clock is not known, but it responds to many of the same environmental factors as the circadian clock: nutritional status, social factors, and stress. Even melatonin, known to be important in the reproduction of some vertebrates, which can entrain the suprachiasmatic nucleus, has been suggested. Other clocks exist; menstrual synchrony is an example.[82,83] Adolescence is a turbulent time. Hormonal, emotional and sexual changes may result in, or may simply accompany, neurological and psychological alterations. For what it is worth, total sleep time in adolescence (boys and girls) is decreased and REM latency is reduced in boys as it is in schizophrenia. However, although the p-value for total sleep time is less than 0.001 comparing 13- to 15-year-old boys with 16- to 19-year-old boys, there is no significant difference for girls in the same age groups. There is no significant difference for either gender when REM latency is compared between these groups. Between 16- through 19-year-olds and 20- to 29-year-olds, total sleep time has a p-value of less than 0.05 for girls and less than 0.01 for boys, while REM latency for boys has a p-value of less than 0.01 in these age groups.[84] Not very convincing.

Incidence, prevalence, etiology, twin studies and genetic factors are not relevant to this exposition, although it is obvious they might be, particularly genetic, if more were known. Suffice to say, a variety of factors has been suggested etiologically. Placental environment,[85] mode of delivery, fetal anoxia, viral infections *in utero* or postpartum, nerve cell migrations, reelin, myelin dysregulation,[86] autoimmunity, a bad mother, social stresses, double binds, even cats have been implicated. "First Gene for Social Behavior Identified in Whiskery Mice" writes the New York Times,[87] which then describes the inattention to barbering in mice deprived of the disheveled gene. In addition to asocial behavior, these mice showed an inability to screen out extraneous noise and focus on a single stimulus. The similarity to schizophrenia, with its hyperattentive state and lack of normal social behavior, elicited comment. The disheveled gene is a key component of signaling pathways of the Wnt family of genes which has been indicted in the genesis of schizophrenia[88] as has reelin, a brain protein that modulates synaptic plasticity, stimulates dendritic growth and regulates neuronal migration. Reduced expression of reelin has been found in schizophrenia.[89,90] Of greater immediate pertinence is the issue of neurotransmitters in both the understanding and the treatment of the syndromes. Of the five types of dopamine receptors, D_2 appears to be the important one in the treatment of schizophrenia. The conventional antipsychotics block D_2 receptors and work well in about two-thirds of the patients with positive symptoms. Newer "atypical" antipsychotics block receptors for serotonin, acetycholine and histamine. By knowing the transmitter, we can locate cell groups and identify (or at least postulate) a role in symptom production.

Clinically, the schizophrenias have been divided into three types of symptoms: positive, negative, or cognitive. Positive symptoms are associated with excess dopamine and negative symptoms with a deficit of dopamine.[91] Perhaps these are not three types of a single illness, but three distinct diseases with three different mechanisms of production. The unifying factors in all three are disturbance of mood, thinking and behavior, although the separation of thinking and behavior is really not possible by an observer, since what another individual thinks is determined by overt behavior. However, thought disorder may be manifested in speech, writing, and art (all of which are behavior), particularly as neologistic, cryptic, idiosyncratic, disconnected speech known as word salad.

The positive symptoms are an exaggeration of phenomena that, normally occur: (1) abnormalities of perception including hallucinations; (2) abnormalities of inferential thinking including delusion; (3) abnormalities of speech presumably reflecting disorganization of ideas and (4) inappropriate behavior indicative of abnormal control. In contrast, the negative symptoms reflect the decrease or absence of phenomenon that normally occur: (1) a decrease in goal-directed behavior — avolition; (2) a decrease in emotional expression called "blunting of affect"; (3) decreased fluency alleged to reflect a decrease of ideas and (4) lack of attention to the environment.[92] Two points follow: (1) Despite his historical influence on psychiatric thinking, Jackson's ideas of positive and negative effects of neurological lesions do not apply to positive and negative symptoms of schizophrenia, though it has been suggested that "The psychotism factor may represent release phenomena in which higher integrative centers are no longer in control",[93] while negative symptoms are the product of "a more diffuse neural loss". Negative neurological lesions, that is the loss or destruction of tissue, may produce negative symptoms but cannot produce positive effects. When positive symptoms appear with neurological lesions, they are released. Lower regions of the nervous system are uninhibited, freed to become evident. Usually, the quality of the released positive neurological phenomena differs from the normal. In schizophrenia, the positive and negative symptoms differ from the norm in quantity and amplitude, as if the volume of an audio receiver or the brightness of a video receiver had been turned up or turned down. (2) The expressed positivity or negativity gives no information about the positivity or negativity of the underlying process. The apathetic, disinterested, non-participatory negative patient may be expressing negative symptoms representing a negative process or may be expressing negative symptoms that reflect an extremely overactive process; a process so overactive that it produces a hyperalertness and information overload that can be handled only by ignoring it, by closing down the motor expression, or hyperactivity of an inhibitory neural mechanism which causes shutdown of behavioral expression. Conclusions about the process, the production mechanism of symptoms, cannot be inferred (however tempting it may be) from the symptoms. How else could we understand the contemporaneous expression of positive and negative symptoms in some patients? Negative symptoms and may be a prodrome to positive symptoms and may be present simultaneously, or may appear after positive symptoms have remitted,[94] without the implication they are the negative of the positive symptoms — a burnout.

Catatonia, less frequent than in the past, can be classified as a negative symptom or can be considered as a separate entity in part because one form is accompanied by excitement. Karl Ludwig Kahlbaum, who originated the term "catatonia" wrote, "These cases…show all the additional signs of mania, such as flight of ideas, agitation, etc."[95] More usually, however, it appears as "a brain disease…in which the mental symptoms are consecutively: melancholy, mania, stupor, confusion and eventually dementia…".

"In addition to the mental symptoms, locomotor — neural processes with the general character of convulsions occur as typical symptoms".[95] Although it is often emphasized that for accuracy of diagnosis, the mood disorder must precede the motor abnormality in psychiatric catatonia, it is the motor aspect that is most striking. The striatum is a key structure regulating movement and has long been postulated as a factor in schizophrenia.[96] Without citing data, Jelliffe writes in 1927 of "Extensive alterations in the basal ganglia…in certain schizophrenic (catatonic) patients".[97] Its role in catatonia is suggested by observations of low levels of striatal dopamine in neuroleptic naïve catatonic patients.[98] The motor signs of catatonic stupor appear in other disorders of striatum such as Parkinson's disease as well as in metabolic or toxic disorders, subfrontal or interhemispheric abnormalities, and even as a complication of neuroleptic medication.[99]

In schizophrenia, the disturbance of mood, thinking and behavior takes place in the presence of a clear sensorium, distinguishing schizophrenia from encephalopathies — either of toxic, metabolic, infectious, or degenerative type. The cognitive disorder may merge into the other two types, but for purposes of classification it is well-advised to treat it separately. Thought disorder is present despite intact formal intelligence. In general, orientation is intact and memory is good, although both orientation and memory may be hard to test. But there is misinterpretation of reality. There may be confusion of parts for wholes, difficulty in separating relevant from irrelevant, parcellation of thoughts and reconstruction in illogical ways, condensation of separate items, circumstantiality and tangentiality as well as distortion of conceptual relationships. "Often there is a tendency to be overinclusive rather than to miss the features of a stimulus."[100]

Positive symptoms imply occurrences beyond normal experience. Agitation, paranoid ideation, hallucinations — usually auditory, delusions, and idée fixe may appear. Mistrust, hostility, aloofness, suspicion, resentment, coldness, ideas of reference, litigiousness, persecutory delusions, grandiose religiosity, hypochondriasis (including being dead), well-organized, illogical insistence all occur. Classical antipsychotic medications provide some relief for patients with positive symptoms. Negative symptoms respond less well. They are emotional withdrawal with blunted affect, loss of interest in the environment, catatonia or other movement disorder. Lack of eye blinking or of the associated movement of arm swing is reminiscent of Parkinson's disease as is the echolalia, echopraxia and stereotypy of catatonia. Even catalepsy has been reported, as are periods of anorexia and insomnia, suggesting hypothalamic and activating system participation. Catatonia also appears in a restless excited form in contrast to the more usual mute negativism with posturing and apparent stupor despite awareness of surroundings. How reminiscent catatonia is of postencephalitic Parkinsonism and like Parkinson's disease, it responds to treatment with selegiline.[101]

Widespread brain dysfunction, as determined by paper and pencil tests,[102] and the ability to form new memories may be impaired. Perception is altered if one is to judge from schizophrenic art but this perspective is apt to be risky when orangutan paintings are fetching high prices without the implication that the painting represents what the ape sees; or even that Cubism represented what Picasso saw. But there is substantial evidence that perception is altered in schizophrenia. "The physical distortions of the external world in schizophrenics is considerably greater than is generally realized…almost all of them (the patients) had fairly marked perceptual disturbances (e.g. 'the floor seems to tilt', 'objects look sort of wavy', 'voices fade and get louder')".[103] Shown an illuminated lightbulb, 75% of 100 non-psychotic controls saw white, silver or yellow. In contrast only 53.3% of 90 schizophrenics (before the days of phenothiazines) saw the expected colors.[103] Mettler writes, "Throughout the history of psychiatry…distortions in perception are a constant feature of clinical descriptions. Among the most frequently mentioned of these are extra-auricular auditory phenomena (hearing with the elbow, kneecap, etc.) sudden bursting and crackling sensations in the head, distortions in perspective, depersonalization of parts of the somatesthetically important parts of the body, and other, less commonly encountered disturbances, many of which may be occasionally experienced by nonpsychotic individuals as a result of acknowledged organic neurologic lesions or toxic or febrile states."[104] In addition, schizophrenic patients report distortion of vision.[105]

Also reported are: (1) abnormal field dependence — Witkin's finding in schizophrenic women — indicates a fragmentation of visual perception due to heightened attention and consists of an inability to extract distinctive features; (2) difficulty with spatial orientation; (3) loss of constancy in perception of size, shape, and distance; (4) flattening or tilting of the visual world; (5) raised threshold for perception of motion; (6) emphasis on details of visual form with less attention to the total picture — really another manifestation of increased field dependence; (7) difficulty shifting attention which may represent overactivity of the attention–arousal system which becomes "overfocused" when activity is heightened; (8) distorted perception of the body. The literature for these observations is listed in Ref. 106. It is said that the visual perceptual difficulties appear early in schizophrenia and predict the severity and course of the disorder.

Blunting or heightening of sensation is reported:[103] Sounds are too loud or a shout becomes a whisper; colors are too bright, a touch may be painful. It is as if a gain setting system was not functioning at the proper level. The lower raphé nuclei and magnocellular portions of the reticular formation, especially the gigantocellular reticular nucleus, and the coeruleus–subcoeruleus complex serve as part of a level setting system widely distributed in brain stem. When the gain is set too high, too much information gets in, which accounts for the fact that there is a tendency to be overinclusive. Schizophrenics report they cannot control what they notice[104] and heightened general arousal has been demonstrated by galvanic skin resistance.[105]

Normal perception is largely visual because it is spatial. It is only in vision that the perception of multiple features occurs simultaneously. It could be argued that there is a spatial aspect to smell and to taste, as they are composed of multiple fragrances that must be perceived at the same moment, but this is rather different from vision, as is somatic sensation, despite its spatial summation. Vision offers a multitude of input stimuli from which distinctive features must be extracted to form a percept. This is the difficulty separating the relevant from the irrelevant, noted as a symptom of schizophrenia. Too much visual information is getting in and serves as the stimulus for behavior, which, if verbal, becomes a stimulus for more verbalization. The visual requires light so the schizophrenic talks more in the light than in the dark just as birds sing with the coming of daylight. In patients, this may not result from visual imagery (although visual imagery is often included in the speech content), but rather indicate visual non-image forming immediate alerting aspect of light ascribed to posterior thalamus and cortex.[4] Some years ago, we did a study in which the talk time in the light was compared to talk time in the dark, six periods of five minutes each alternated a light and totally dark environment (Figs. 8, 9). The dependence of schizophrenics on visual stimuli is demonstrated by their 30% dark–light talk time ratio compared with 100% for aphasics and 110% for dements. The talk was often about the visual environment and would become disjointed, stimulated by an uttered word. Speech served as an auditory percept which stimulated the same or similar sounding speech without reference to the meaning.[109]

"You meet and start getting gold on both sides. Two noses. Well no mast glass. I took that last wing past last night. But they might be sold for old gold no matter which way I go". says Hazel, a patient.

The hyperattentiveness, confirmed by hypermetabolic cortical positron emission studies,[110] is not limited to visual percepts. Non-linguistic sounds also intrude. An automobile horn honked outside the hospital and a moment later, the word honking appeared in a semantically irrelevant manner. A plane flew overhead — a sound the average Bostonian ignores and never hears — and Hazel started to sing, "Coming in on a wing and a prayer" (a World War II song). I can't help but wonder in retrospect if the "wing" in the paragraph

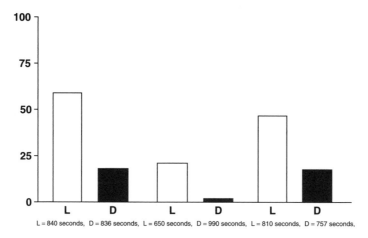

L = 840 seconds, D = 836 seconds, L = 650 seconds, D = 990 seconds, L = 810 seconds, D = 757 seconds,

Fig. 8. Dark:Light. Ordinate in percent. Open bar (L) percent spontaneous speech in light. Closed bar (D) percent spontaneous speech in dark. Each pair of bars represents a different schizophrenic patient.

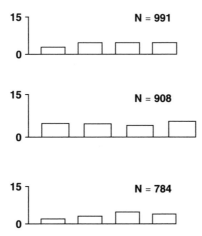

Fig. 9. Frequency of repetition of similar sounding words. N represents the total number of words in the sample. Ordinate is expressed in percent of total sample. Abscissa from left to right represents the first through fourth positions following each word in the sample. Each display represents an individual schizophrenic patient.

above ("Last wing past last") was a plane that hyperattentive Hazel heard and I did not.

Other examples of the visual trigger:

1. Hazel walks into the room and starts talking about "epalsy," staring straight at *Epilepsy Abstracts.*
2. She spells out the title of *Journal of Comparative Neurology* which is in her visual field.
3. She speaks of having "lunch in a *comparatively* small hole".
4. When asked the date, she gives the date printed on the cover of the *Journal of Comparative Neurology.*
5. Two lamps were very close together having been moved to make room for the recording equipment. Hazel said, "You left both lamps hugging too much".
6. During the conversation, I closed my eyes and she speaks of "sleepy hollow".
7. She refers to Worcester and to wisteria. The *Journal of Comparative Neurology* was issued by the "Wistar Institute", the name of which is on the cover.
8. The Directory of the Departments of Anatomy, similar in appearance to the *Journal of Comparative Neurology,* was substituted between sessions. In the second session, references to the Directory of the Departments of Anatomy occur.[109]

This hyperattentive visual state is explored in the study by Witkin and colleagues,[111] which examined the perception of a mobile framed rod in relation to the vertical by patients seated in a tiltable chair in a room which could be moved from plumb to 56 degrees. Eight of ten paranoid schizophrenic women were influenced by the prevailing field as were control women. In contrast, seven of 12 paranoid schizophrenic men were relatively uninfluenced by field. It should come as no surprise that the vestibular system is not a better indicator in this study (bodily sensation is compensated for by rotating the room around a track of 22 feet in diameter), when for most of us during flight takeoff, the impression is usually that the plane is level and the ground is tilted.

In 1933, Paul Schilder discusses the relation between the vestibular apparatus and perception in psychosis.[60] He notes that there is a difference between a peripheral and a central lesion. There is apparent movement not entirely dependent on nystagmus, with transformation from one plane to another. Polyopia and micropsia, homolateral to a central vestibular lesion are also noted. The postural model of the body is under vestibular influence. Heaviness and lightness or dissociation of a body part may occur. Perceptual changes are often induced by motion so the patient may limit movement. It is suggested that catatonic immobility may ensue.[112] Changes are incorporated into delusional experience or hallucinations. A number of patients note rotation, spinning, relation to movement. There is a report of a patient made dizzy by sounds. One of my patients reported a buzzing — a machine recording her voice — that made her dizzy.[109] In addition to these perceptual changes, there are changes in muscle tone.

Abnormality of eye movement is prominent in schizophrenia as it is in Parkinson's disease and implies abnormality of the vestibular system, which has an intimate connection by way of the medial longitudinal bundle with the oculomotor nuclei of the brain stem. Eye movement abnormality in schizophrenia has long been known. Inaccurate pursuit was described in 1908.[113] In addition, saccadic movement, spontaneous or reduced nystagmus, vestibuloocular reflex and optokinetic nystagmus should be evaluated.[114] Abnormality may represent a problem with motor control, sensory input or attention. The vestibular system plays an important role in each. "Motor control over most eye movements appeared to be normal in schizophrenic patients: They are able to generate slow and fast eye movements (such as nystagmus) in response to vestibular stimulation. Full-field optokinetic responses as well as oculocephalic reflex are intact; and both latency and accuracy of voluntary saccades essentially normal. Only SPEM (smooth pursuit eye movements) generated when pursuing a moving target are impaired in schizophrenic patients."[115]

Assessment of vestibular function in schizophrenics, as in all humans, must be limited to evaluation of specific function for there is no way to evaluate vestibular contribution to the arousal mechanism independent of other sensory input. All modalities have lost their markers prior to arrival at the activating system so are indistinguishable, one from the other. The usual appraisable of specific vestibular function is by eye movements. Such studies which cannot implicate unambiguously the vestibular system because of the inclusion of motor and other sensory mechanisms, employs the stepping test. In this procedure, the blind-folded subject is made to march 50 steps in place with arms extended forward. The normal individual completes the test pointing in the same direction as from the start; the patient with vestibular imbalance manifests angular deviation (rotation or displacement). One study[116] demonstrated abnormality in 73 of 82 schizophrenic patients, indicating "highly possible involvement of the vestibular system in schizophrenia". Slight hyperactivity of the level of synchronization between left and right vestibular nuclei has been reported.[117]

To test the postulate that the schizophrenic patient is hyperalert (that is, the arousal system is overactive), the access route, in addition to clinical observation, is to assess the attentional mechanism, with the implication that attention is an indicator of activation. Focused attention with inhibition of irrelevant stimuli is impaired in schizophrenia,[118–122] the usual manifestation of which is intrusion of irrelevant stimuli to awareness. This suggests a hyperattentive state, or at least insufficient suppresion of ambient attention, preventing adequate focus.

Before assessing the role of vestibular function in schizophrenia, an important consideration needs to be reiterated. What if, as Bleuler indicated, schizophrenia is not a single disease. It is not even a group of separate diseases that look alike. On clinical grounds, catatonia is very different from paranoia. On chemical grounds, schizophrenia with negative symptoms which respond poorly to conventional antipsychotics is different from schizophrenia with positive symptoms that respond much more favorably. Selegiline, used in the treatment of Parkinson's disease, is being used with some success for negative symptoms. It is a wake-up drug, a monoamine oxidase B inhibitor, with partial conversion to amphetamine. As a wake-up drug, it must work somewhere on the reticular activating system, perhaps to compensate for decreased vestibular input. Suppose the vestibular symptoms are overactive in the delusional, hallucinatory patient and deficient in the rigid, immobile, echolalic Parkinsonian-like catatonic. Reports on eye movements, or on the vestibular system, which do not distinguish the nature of the schizophrenic patients in a cohort, can only be used with caution, if at all. The citation in Ornitz[112] of five reports — all before the advent of the phenothiazines which may affect vestibular response — of at least 36 catatonic patients with absent or diminished nystagmus in response to caloric or rotary stimulation (or both) suggests, as postulated, decreased activity somewhere along the vestibular pathways. The fact that caloric, rotational or galvanic stimulation does not evoke a response does not mean the defect is in the labyrinth, although it does not exclude it. In patients in whom the clinical state fluctuates, the vestibular reactivity parallels the clinical state, which alternates between stupor and relative freedom from symptoms.[123] Other studies of unselected schizophrenic patients[124] for example, showed mixed results because I suspect, they studied mixed patients. An old study, done before the advent of phenothiazines, seems particularly important.[125] Thirteen schizophrenic patients, of whom four were catatonic, underwent caloric and galvanic vestibular testing. Impairment of vestibular response was found only in the catatonic patients. Two, who were in the midst of a catatonic period, had complete absence of response. A third, at the onset of a period of catatonia, had a hypoactive response, as did the fourth, who was at the end of a period of catatonia. It is unfortunate that a given patient could not be followed longitudinally through a catatonic cycle. However, if one constructs a hypothetical time line, placing one patient at the beginning, one at the end and two in the middle, it suggests that in catatonia vestibular depression comes on slowly, reaches a maximum of complete dysfunction and then with a waning of symptoms, recovers. Several speculative implications follow: (1) Whatever the process, it is dynamic, not static. It progresses and regresses so it is not destructive of structure. In a patient in whom the clinical state fluctuates, the vestibular reactivity parallels the clinical state which alternates between stupor and freedom from symptoms.[126] (2) Its location is not evident from the experimental setup, but it appears likely to be located in the end-organ or first nuclear waystation. (3) Efferent input to the semicircular canals has been demonstrated. (4) Vestibular efferents arise widely in brain stem reticular formation. (5) Vestibular efferents can modify the gain of vestibular afferents. (6) Increased arousal, generated by brain stem reticular formation, increases vestibular nystagmus produced by caloric stimulation,[123] so presumably decreased arousal or inhibitory feedback to vestibular efferents could diminish a vestibular afferent response. (7) Selegiline, used in the treatment of catatonia, increases the availability of monoaminergic transmitters. It would be of interest to determine its effect on caloric nystagmus in catatonia. The finding of absent caloric nystagmus at the height of the catatonic episode is compatible with the postulate of an overactive reticular activating system; an example would be overactivity of gigantocellular reticular nucleus, from which vestibular efferents arise, and which contains inhibitory glycinergic neurons. In this instance, the hyperactivity would be an inhibitory component expressing itself through the vestibular efferent effect on vestibular afferent response to caloric stimulation.

Smooth pursuit has been studied during caloric stimulation in actively psychotic patients compared with outpatient schizophrenics and normal controls. Failure of visual fixation to suppress caloric nystagmus was related to disordered tracking before and after caloric stimulation. Dysrhythmia and reduced fast phase velocity of nystagmus also occurred in the group.[127] Surprisingly, the outpatient schizophrenics in remission did not show this abnormality, surprising because 25–40% of asymptomatic first-degree relatives of schizophrenics show impaired smooth pursuit eye movements which resemble deficits seen in patients with lesions of what are called middle temporal and medial superior temporal regions of the motion-sensitive areas of the parietal lobe.[115] However, single photon emission tomography locates the abnormality in the right and left superior prefrontal area and left inferior prefrontal cortex, as well as the left anterior and posterior cingulate.[128] Saccadic performance is allegedly controlled by four cortical areas: posterior parietal, frontal eye fields, supplementary eye fields and dorsolateral prefrontal cortex with caudate, cerebellum and superior colliculus included in the circuitry. In schizophrenics (five paranoid, seven disorganized, 17 undifferentiated and one residual), the abnormality was consistent with the dysfunction of the dorsolateral prefrontal cortex, the caudate or both.[129] Caloric testing in 12 schizophrenic patients on phenothiazines for more than one month revealed some depression of response "in nearly half".[130] The uncertainty may result from the dissociation of past pointing, nystagmus, vertigo and vegetative reactions, all of which were assessed. The problem, as the author of this study acknowledges, is that schizophrenic patients tested before the advent of phenothiazines also showed a hypoactive tendency.

If, as postulated,[131] optokinetic nystagmus is composed of pursuit and saccades, it makes sense to study optokinetic nystagmus in schizophrenics because of their known pursuit impairment. One problem is that it is virtually impossible nowadays to find schizophrenic patients who have not received phenothiazines or similar drugs. Before the era of drug therapy, optokinetic nystagmus testing was uncommon. So in any assessment, the effect of drugs must be taken into account. When cortical and subcortical optokinetic nystagmus are tested separately, full-field (subcortical) optokinetic nystagmus is normal (33 schizophrenics, type unspecified, all but two on antipsychotic medication, only five of whom underwent full-field examination), but partial-field (cortical) optokinetic nystagmus is impaired, the slow phase of the nystagmus demonstrating dysrhythmia.[132] This implies that the "Cortex does exact some inhibitory function over vestibular response".[103] This is confirmed in a study in which full-field optokinetic nystagmus was not impaired in schizophrenics in whom partial-field optokinetic nystagmus was abnormal. Full-field optokinetic nystagmus stabilizes the visual field when the subject is in motion. Partial-field optokinetic nystagmus stabilizes the moving object, but not the full-field. With the former comes a sense of rotation; with the latter, subjective rotation does not occur. Full-field optokinetic nystagmus reflects subcortical mechanisms; it persists following the decortication. The pathway is allegedly retina, optic tract, lateral geniculate body, cerebellum, vestibular nuclei integrated in the paramedian pontine reticular formation. Partial-field optokinetic nystagmus consists of cortical projection to pontine reticular formation where it joins projections from the full-field pathways.

Perhaps the most interesting report in schizophrenia was limited to the study of cortical optokinetic nystagmus. One hundred and eighteen patients were diagnosed as dementia praecox and 73 patients as chronic hallucinatory; presumably, all were on medication. If the patients with the diagnosis of dementia praecox are to be understood as having negative symptoms and the hallucinatory patients as having positive symptoms, the results are of great importance for the optokinetic nystagmus is more severely disturbed in the dementia praecox than in the hallucinatory patients.[133] We observed impairment of optokinetic nystagmus in nine out of 12 patients with tardive dyskinesia.[134] A matched control group of schizophrenic patients on medication revealed normal optokinetic nystagmus in 12 of 13 and the abnormality of optokinetic nystagmus in tardive dyskinesia has been reported by others.[71]

The abnormality of eye movement in non-psychotic first-degree relatives of schizophrenics needs further scrutiny. It clearly indicates that psychosis and eye movement abnormality are separable. This may be because they are produced by two separate systems. The eye movement abnormality may be an epiphenomenon, which occurs in only about 25 to 40% of the first-degree relatives and in only 40 to 80% of the schizophrenics, so it is not a requirement in psychosis. Both the eye movement abnormality and the psychosis may be produced by the same system, but at different locations; the eye movement abnormality by the specific input of the vestibular system — either end-organ or nuclear — and the psychosis by nonspecific input to the activating system. In this construct, the psychosis-producing aspect would need amplification in the reticular formation for the positive symptoms or dampening for the negative ones. Or a third possible formulation is that both eye signs and psychosis are a manifestation of output alteration at the initial stage of input where the balance between the two sides, whether the end-organ signal is heightened or depressed for positive or negative symptoms respectively, is equal, so there are no eye signs, or nearly equal, so the eye signs are mild. The heightened or depressed input to the reticular formation generates, without the need for amplification or depression, the hyperalert state of the positive form or the apathetic, disinterested negative disorder. Many of the reported symptoms suggest initiation early in vestibular input — tilt, wavy, dizzy, apparent movement and perceptual changes induced by motion. That this may not be so is suggested in the normal by the immediate but quickly compensated effect of new (usually stronger) prescription glasses; the world may seem tipped, there may be dizziness, and the terror of going down a flight of stairs is increased by movement.

Directional preponderance is yet another measure of vestibular function. Tonic output from the vestibular nuclei is paralleled by tonic output from temporal lobe which is fed back to the vestibular nuclei. Together, these maintain the symmetry of nystagmus to caloric stimulation. Normally, the duration of nystagmus in each direction is the same, that is, left and right ear with hot irrigation and left and right ear with cold irrigation. In the presence of a temporal lobe lesion, a directional preponderance reflecting the decline of temporal tonic output occurs (toward the side of the lesion). Eighteen of 50 chronic schizophrenics (before the advent of neuroleptic therapy) showed directional preponderance. In 16 of the 18, the directional preponderance of the slow component was to the left.[110]

The role of the vestibular aparatus in schizophrenia has been explored in a study of motion perception. The argument is based on the relationship between the perception of movement across the retina and the presence of a comparator, an efference copy, generated by eye movements. When they match, there is no perception of movement. When they differ, movement is noted. Movement threshold depends upon the detectability of this difference. The efference copy generated by eye movement is intimately related to the vestibular system. If the vestibular system is noisy, the threshold should be elevated, and so it was found to be in schizophrenia.[135] Once again, the type of schizophrenia was not specified, but if the predominance was of positive symptoms, this would fit well with the argument for an overactive vestibular system in one form of the disorder. The notion of the efference copy has been expanded since this study,[136] but the general conclusion remains unaltered.

Where the abnormality occurs in the vestibular system is not evident. One possibility is that it is in the nonspecific components, a possibility considered in the discussion of the arousal system. A second possibility is affection of the specific projections to the cortex. A third option is that it relates to the connections with cerebellum, a structure associated with overreaction or under-reaction to stimuli.[137] If it is generated early, say in the vestibular nuclei, it could be in all locations. Attempts to assign a given area in the brain the responsibility for producing schizophrenia's symptoms, either negative or less likely, positive, implies a static conception of the organization of the nervous system and of the psyche. A dynamic view is preferable and does not preclude the participation of systems and their components. For example, the suggestion that striatal dysfunction produces perceptual disorder similar to that observed in schizophrenia and that "schizophrenic individuals may suffer from a striatal dysfunction"[96] does not place schizophrenia in the striatum; it also allows for consideration of the projections of the vestibular system to the substantia nigra then to the striatum by way of the pallidum, to the vestibular cortex.[138] Pallidal damage "may be so severe as to present an appearance reminiscent of *flexibilitas cerea.*"[104]

Just as eye movement can be used to explore the specific contribution of the vestibular system to schizophrenia, sleep can be used to explore the vestibular contribution to the nonspecific system, although the distinction from other sensory input is not as clear as in the case of eye movement. However, a rich reciprocal connection exists between the vestibular nuclei and the reticular formation, allowing speculation about the role of vestibular input in the sleep of the schizophrenic.

As Parkinson noted in his patients, so does Bleuler in his. "In schizophrenia, sleep is habitually disturbed."[81] In general terms, the disturbance can be characterized as profound insomnia, often appearing as a prodromal symptom, long-sleep onset latency and reduced total sleep time with frequent wakenings as if the arousal gain is set too high. However, these comments are based on studies that did not distinguish between patients with positive symptoms and patients with negative symptoms and often the medication status is not controlled or not stated — a point of potential importance as first-generation antipsychotics increase total sleep time and sleep efficiency (defined as the ratio of time asleep to time in bed) and reduce sleep latency and nocturnal wakings. Second-generation antipsychotics have the same effects on total sleep time, sleep latency, sleep efficiency and nocturnal wakings. They also, if clozapine can be taken as representative, increase Stage 2 sleep and reduce Stage 4 sleep in schizophrenia compared to a medication-free period. REM time is unchanged in comparison with normals, whether the patient is having hallucinations or not. Of interest is the relation of the decreased REM latency of unmedicated schizophrenics to normal controls. Half the studies reported decreased REM latency in patients; even in the studies that found no difference between patients and controls, a bimodal distribution of REM latency was disclosed among schizophrenics. One cannot help but wonder about the relation to positive and negative symptoms. Abnormalities of Stage 4 time or amplitude have been reported. As a generalization, positive symptoms correlate with increased REM sleep eye movement density (the ratio of eye movement frequency to REM sleep time), which could be interpreted as increased vestibular activity. Positive symptoms also include short REM latency, reduced sleep efficiency and increased sleep latency which correlates with cerebrospinal fluid-orexin levels in schizophrenia.[139] Negative symptoms correlate with a deficiency of slow-wave sleep[140–142] and increased delta sleep correlates with an improvement of negative symptoms.[143] Shortened REM sleep latency and slow-wave sleep deficit was not found in 22 drug-naïve paranoid schizophrenics (i.e., with positive symptomatology), just prolonged sleep onset latency, increased wake time and decreased Stage 2 sleep, all compatible with an active or overactive arousal system.[144]

Finally, a reduction of sleep spindles in schizophrenia is reported. Twelve subjects were diagnosed as paranoid, two as disorganized and four as residual. All were on medication and were compared with normals and with depressed patients. A reduction of sleep spindle number, amplitude, duration and integrated activity that allowed a greater than 90% discrimination between schizophrenia and the other groups was found.[141] Ordinarily, sleep spindles occur in Stage 2 sleep. However, they can also occur, in REM sleep.[145] They are generated by a thalamocortical circuit which is influenced by brain stem input. The reticular cholinergic system has a dampening effect on spindle genesis and the reticular neurons that project to intralaminar thalamus stop discharging about one second before the appearance of a spindle sequence during stage transition period. "The withdrawal of tonic brainstem reticular discharges is probably an effective factor for spindle genesis at two thalamic targets."[146] What this means is that spindle suppression in schizophrenia indicates a reticular formation that is more active than in normal controls — activity that conceivably relates to an increased vestibular input.

Two interesting observations should be mentioned in a discussion of the relations among vestibular function, schizophrenia and REM sleep. It has been shown[147] that following REM deprivation, schizophrenics in remission showed a marked increase of REM sleep time in comparison to acutely ill schizophrenics who did not show even an expected normal increase. Alteration of eye movement density during REM sleep has also been noted. This is alleged to be mediated by spontaneous activity of the vestibular "centers" (end-organ, nuclei or other location not specified) and is paralleled by the reduction of nystagmus to induced vestibular activity (method of stimulation not specified: caloric, rotation, galvanic) in awake schizophrenics.[112] It has been shown that the medial and the descending vestibular nuclei discharge at high frequency during REM[148] and that bilateral destruction of these nuclei eliminates REM.[149]

This, of course, implies that the vestibular system is less active in acute schizophrenia than in the compensated patient — a finding that would be at odds with the prediction, unless all patients exhibited only negative symptoms — an unlikely possibility. However, if the distinction between the specific and non-specific input is borne in mind, an explanation is at hand. Eye movement implies an imbalance, however brief, of vestibular specific input whether for REM sleep or waking gaze. Alertness or arousal implies a heightened vestibular input of the nonspecific system, whether balanced or not. Eye movement and arousal can be affected separately by vestibular input so REM sleep eye movements do not constitute an accurate measure of the state of reticular activation.

Instead of sleep, another approach would be to consider the pharmacologic effects of drugs known to stimulate the reticular activating system and also cause schizophrenic-like symptoms. Amphetamine, which stimulates dopamine release, mimics the positive symptoms of schizophrenia and phencyclidine (angel dust) mimics the negative and cognitive (and at times, the positive) symptoms. Therefore, we might predict that amphetamine would stimulate and phencyclidine depress the brain stem activating system.

In man, amphetamine, produces an increase in wake time, more so for the dextro-isomer than for the levo, and both forms reduce desynchronized sleep.[150] Amphetamines also reduce sleep efficiency, increase the number of awakenings and decrease Stage 2 (spindle stage), slow wave and REM sleep similar to findings in schizophrenia. "Ecstasy", a potent hallucinogens, is methamphetamine with an additional dimethoxy ring; other hallucinogens have been created by variations on the basic amphetamine structure. Amphetamine and its derivatives enhance the release and inhibit the reuptake of dopamine and norepinephrine. Ascending dopamine projections arise in the mesencephalic ventral tegmental area as well as the substantia nigra. A pathway from the substantia nigra terminates in the dorsal striatum. A second pathway from the ventral tegmental area and the medial substantia nigra projects to the anterior cingulate gyrus, as well as the medial prefrontal and entorhinal areas. These cortical areas communicate with the ventral tegmental area and the nucleus accumbens. Glutamate is the transmitter and when dopamine release is increased from the ventral tegmental area into the nucleus accumbens, the responsiveness of the accumbens and the ventral tegmental area to glutamate is altered for days.[151] The projection from the ventral tegmental area is involved in electrographic arousal.[152] Psychiatric symptoms as a result of amphetamine are usually dose-dependent, but chronic use of low dose, or a single high dose, may produce psychosis. Paranoid delusions, blunted affect, motor tics, and perseveration occur.[153] An interesting speculative point relates to the heightened response predicated in schizophrenia. Sensitization to amphetamine follows abstinence. One postulate relates to delta FosB, a stable protein that lasts for months after amphetamine use. Delta FosB may be responsible for increasing dendritic spines on noradrenergic neurons, causing amplification of symptoms between cells.[151]

Phencyclidine, like the anesthetic ketamine, does not require prolonged use to create its effect. Brief low doses of either can produce the negative symptoms of schizophrenia. These agents apparently exercise their effects on the glutamine transmitter systems. Glutamine is the main excitatory transmitter in brain. A receptor known as the N-methyl-D-aspartate (NMDA) glutamate receptor is blocked by these drugs. Dopamine release is partly controlled by the NMDA receptor and is disturbed with blockade by phencyclidine or ketamine. "Glutamate synthesizing neurons comprise the projection neurons of the reticular formation, thalamus and cerebral cortex and are thus critical at all levels in the process of cortical activation."[154] So the agents that depress brain stem reticular formation by depressing glutamate function produce motor slowing, reduced speech and withdrawals, the negative symptoms of schizophrenia, and by way of alteration of dopamine release, can produce positive symptoms of schizophrenia. NMDA receptors are thought to strengthen connections between neurons and to participate in gain control or level setting. The hyperattentive state of the paranoid or hallucinating schizophrenic could be a manifestation of a gain set too high while the apathetic non-participation of catatonia could reflect a gain set too low. To speculate, the eye movement abnormalities in schizophrenics, may be a faulty input by the vestibular system, either too much to set the level too high or too little to cause rigid catatonia.

What can be learned from imaging studies? It is always risky to equate structure and function for either may be disturbed without affection of the other. However, form often follows function in the developing brain and one theory of schizophrenia is that is an adult life expression of a fetal abnormality, perhaps related to reelin, a protein in brain that regulates cell migration, stimulates dendrite production and enhances long-term potentiation. Failure of normal synaptic pruning during adolescence has been postulated.[155] Imaging has shown a wide distribution of changes. Increase of ventricular size, cerebellar changes (particularly in the vermis), cortical loss in childhood, decreased size of the hippocampus and the amygdala, reduction in size of the inferior parietal lobe particularly on the left in schizophrenic men, left posterior temporal gyrus reduction,[156] and changes in the right and left prefrontal, left inferior prefrontal, anterior and posterior cingulate[128] are all noted. In discordant identical twins, the schizophrenic twin had a smaller hippocampus and larger ventricles, including the third, in contrast to monozygotic twins without schizophrenia.[157] Unfortunately, handedness and whether some were "mirror twins" was not noted. Medial temporal limbic structures were smaller at postmortem in schizophrenic patients who had never received neuroleptics and changes were atrophic with no gliosis that would suggest infection.[110] Two-thirds showed abnormal sulcal-gyral patterns and one-third had abnormal cytoarchitecture of limbic structures.

The frequent report of ventricular enlargement in schizophrenia must be used with caution. Ventricular enlargement may be primary, a result of hydrocephalus resulting from inadequate spinal fluid drainage, or it may be secondary — so-called hydrocephalus *ex vacuo*, the result of tissue loss. To be useful in an analysis of the causation of schizophrenia, tissue loss must occur first, whereas with primary hydrocephalus, tissue loss may be a result. CT measurements of tissue density help in the distinction so that a loss of tissue density, particularly in the dominant frontal region in the left hemisphere, including monozygotic twins discordant for schizophrenia, is to be noted[110] but with a caveat: The loss of density is more likely to represent fiber loss than cell loss. The fibers come from or go to somewhere else, so loss of density may represent loss of input or loss of output and may indicate disorder elsewhere in the system. The problem with morphologic studies, whether by imaging or by postmortem examination, is determining whether the observed changes are the cause or the effect of the disorder. Even when combined with cognitive tasks[158] or when functional testing (such as eyeblink conditioning) is done with imaging,[159] the problem of cause and effect remains.

Palilalia, echolalia, and echopraxia have always fascinated me. Perhaps mirror neurons are involved. There are mirror neurons responsive to sound — so-called echo neurons, just as there are mirror-neurons responsive to sight. Perhaps they cannot detach from the executive pathways, so the act or the sound is repeated. We all do it all the time, normals less often, dements more frequently. Catatonics and Parkinsonians, compulsively. What we noted in our study of language in schizophrenics[109] is that repetition is less common in schizophrenics than in aphasics (in whom it is called perseveration) or in dements. The amount of repetition increases from the first to the fourth position after a key word and the frequency of similar sounding words correlates with the dark–light ratio (Fig. 8). The greater the ratio, the greater the number of repetitions and the more prominent they are in the first position after a key word. "The less effective visual stimuli are in releasing speech, the greater and more immediate, the efficacy of self-generated auditory stimuli."[109] It is the self-generated auditory stimuli that accounts for klang association. In the Parkinsonian, the repetition, presumably generated by auditory input, is immediate and exact. In the non-catatonic schizophrenic, it may be delayed and similar but not identical.

"The air force man.....the air force man.....is raping...is raping.....and murdering.....and murdering.....me..........................me" says Lillian.

How to put all of this together? The proposal is as follows:

1. The paranoid hallucinatory schizophrenic manifests a different symptom complex from the withdrawn catatonic.
2. Over-attention with intrusion of irrelevant stimuli characterizes the positive symptomatology.
3. Inattention and immobility, perhaps with other signs reminiscent of Parkinson's disease, are present in the negative form of the disorder.
4. Perceptual difficulties are prominent in the positive group and are largely visual; these often suggest vestibular origin.
5. Eye movement abnormalities are present in both groups.
6. Sleep disorder is particularly present in patients with positive symptoms.
7. Eye movements and their disorder relate intimately to the specific function of the vestibular system.
8. Sleep and its disorders relate to the nonspecific ascending reticular activating system.
9. The vestibular system has significant input to the ascending reticular activating system.
10. Amphetamine, phencyclidine and ketamine, which have effects on the ascending reticular activating system, may mimic schizophrenia in users.
11. Amphetamine, which stimulates the dopaminergic system of the reticular formation, mimics the paranoia of the positive symptomatology and the sleep disorder of this variety of schizophrenia.
12. The negative apathetic immobile form of the disorder is reproduced in the normal by phencyclidine or ketamine by blocking the N-methyl-D-aspartate (NMDA) glutamate receptor, the receptors for the major excitatory transmitter in the brain.

13. The vestibular specific system can affect visual perception not only via its connection with the eyes. If overactive, it may be responsible for the tilt or wave perception or sense of motion reported by some schizophrenics.

14. If overactive, its nonspecific input may generate hyperalertness with the intrusion of stimuli into awareness of the schizophrenic with positive symptomatology.

15. If overactive, it might generate the changes in sleep architecture that have been noted in the positive form of the disorder.

16. If underactive, the decreased level of awareness may correlate with the negative symptoms of emotional withdrawal, blunted affect and loss of interest in the environment.

17. Even muscular rigidity, the extreme form of which is catatonia, may represent deficient vestibular input for vestibulospinal input from the lateral vestibular nuclei by way of a reticulospinal tract mediates preganglionic inhibition of the anterior horn cell. When deficient, rigidity may ensue.

These effects, if vestibular in origin, do not imply an end-organ abnormality. They do, however, imply a fairly low-level abnormality because brain structures such as the medial longitudinal fasciculus, the ocular motor nuclei and the mesencephalic reticular formation are involved. It is unlikely this would represent descending input from cortex or subcortex. At the same time, fairly high levels along the vestibular pathways, for example the striatum and the globus pallidus, could participate in the symptomatology.

Chapter 5

PERCEPTION

The contention that perception is altered in schizophrenia has major implications that demand discussion. Perception is a response of the nervous system to objects and events in the environment. It requires a neural base, but perception itself is psychophysical. It is subjective so its representation of the object or event (for economy, let's refer to both as 'object') is not isomorphic (in any sense of the term) with the object. Perception is to be understood as "a response of living organisms to their environments by way of focused or interpretive recognition of what the environment offers."[111] There are at least two ways of looking at the issue. One assumes that the percept is determined to a large degree by the outside world, unrelated to the contributions of the observer. In the second, the discrepancy between the object as it impinges on the sensory transducers, and what the subject perceives, relates to the accumulated experience of the observer. Different people perceive the same stimulus — let's call it reality — differently. "Differences in modes of perceiving...are related to profound differences among people."[111] People (normal people) vary widely in their manner of perception and, in different situations (at least with respect to the perception of the vertical), vary widely in what they see, how they depend on the visual field and how important bodily input is; these attributes or neurological inputs for a given individual are comparatively stable. But people differ.

The percept is conditioned by previous experience, previous percepts, previous and current emotional states, among many other things. Recall the experiment in which episodic injection of epinephrine determined the character of the subject's response. Memory plays a prominent role in perception and might be included as integral to it, not only for previous percepts against which to compare the current experience, but also for prior emotional responses to previous experiences which can influence the affective aspects of the current percept. In this sense then, percepts are not only subjective, but represent the subject acting on the environment. The perceived environment is not neutral; the observer contributes. It is this kind of operation that lets me see faces in the clouds. This action underlies the distinction between perception and apperception. So-called "projective tests" measure aspects of perception that are not inherent to the stimulus. What the subject reports in tests like the Rorschach or the Thematic Apperception Test is not what is in the ambiguous stimulus, but rather, what the subject brings to the stimulus. While this may reflect an attitude or an emotional state, it is also a neurological function taking place at the moment of reporting. By virtue of this action, it is independent of the sensory aspects of the percept. The reporting may represent the action — the apperception, not the stimulus. The stimulus may be neutral, the apperception, paranoid.

Perception requires the presence of a sensory stimulus, but in the strict sense, percepts are created by the simultaneous presence of more than one sensory (in the neurological meaning) stimulus. Sensory stimuli are unimodal (hot or cold, sharp or dull) and are recognized at a thalamic level. Percepts are multimodal and are appreciated by the cortex. Sensory input is modality marked, but factors other than modality generate the subjective percept. Affective aspects of the stimulus object and of the state of the subject contribute. Level of awareness or consciousness plays a role. This introduces a problem, as attention, consciousness or awareness may be present with or without awareness of the awareness. Behavior in the normal or the schizophrenic may be generated by stimuli which are unrecognized — that is, which cannot be verbalized — but that level of attention or consciousness is operating and contributing to perception. This points up the problem that the outside observer can never know what the subject perceives, only what the subject reports by word or by other behavior.

Perception, by way of all five senses, may be multimodal, but the term most commonly refers to vision where the perceptual construct is spatial. In audition, the percept is temporal; for the other three classical senses, it is not very different from sensation. Just as sensation generates perception, so perception generates conception, which no longer requires the presence of the object or sensory input from the external environment except in so far as the brain is part of the environment. From perception and conception comes action on the stimulating environment to change it in some way and so, to provide new percepts.

Suppose we consider the non-classical senses. Vestibular input, generating a sense of movement or position, is not one of the five senses. Nor is position sense, yet both contribute to perception formed by input of the five classical senses. There is strong interaction between the vestibular and visual systems and what is seen — the visual percept — is strongly influenced by these "non-perceptual systems". The visual percept may be badly distorted, although there is no abnormality of the visual system. At least three non-perceptual systems enter into the formation of the percept: Position and movement, emotion and memory. In addition, arousal or attention (particularly in the sense of unfocused vigilance, which in pathological states such as schizophrenia, may become focused) amplifies or diminishes perception and changes the role of the distinctive features. So for example, to consider perception as a function of the visual system is to miss the point.

Sensory aspects of a percept are modality marked. They are transmitted by tracts or fillets, with each tract subserving a single modality. The modalities remain segregated at a thalamic level, (although there are multimodal cells in the superior colliculus) from which they project to the cortex. Collaterals from the modality marked pathways lose their markers and contribute to the ascending reticular activating system which ultimately serves to "wake up" the cortex. An important contribution comes from vestibular input which is always tonically active. Because it is a null indicator, the total level of activity may not be reported; only the algebraic sum of the activity is appreciated, but the level of activity (not the sum) may be effective in generating nonspecific arousal. So the sense of motion generated by an inactive balanced system or by a hyperactive balanced system may each be zero, but the hyperactive system may contribute to a higher level of vigilance or attention or consciousness, which may, in turn, contribute to the psychophysical interpretation of the multisensory input — the percept.

Action on sensory input entails behavioral inhibition as well as attention. Features that are irrelevant to the issue at hand can be ignored. Attention can be focused and background noise can be discarded or at least suppressed. If everything about an event were attended to, information overload would occur. More importantly, the "meaning" of the event would not be set in relief. This accounts for the notion of distinctive features, first formulated with respect to phonological aspects of language, but then realized to have much broader pertinence. Distinctive features of an experience are what make it what it is. It appears in all perceptual experience. In font design, the designer Frere-Jones says that a font works "by taking the unique feature of [each] letter — its essence, the thing that makes it this letter and not something else — and turning it up as loud as it can go,"[160] but distinctive features vary for each observer and are not entirely an attribute of the stimulus. Interpretation in performing arts, for example, vary because of emphasis of different features. Barrymore's Hamlet is a different character from Olivier's. Pissaro and Cezanne painted the same scene at the same time differently, presumably because each saw it differently. Although the notes on the page are the same for each of us, Bach will never be the same since

Glenn Gould. Interpretation is not perception, but it influences future perception. Apperception is perception of new experience in the context of earlier experience.

In the hyperattentive state, distinctive features may get blurred, attention may be directed to non-distinctive as well as distinctive features. There may be too much information. One way to handle information overload is by clustering or grouping. Confronted with a random display of items, if you can group them, you can control them. A standard bedside test of mental status is to repeat a string of random numbers. The examiner enunciates them at a rate of about one per second in a monotone. The normal response is to repeat seven numbers forward and five numbers backward. If, instead of retaining two, seven, four, nine, three, six, you group them into 27, 49, 36, you may be able to repeat seven pairs or 14 numbers. Or look at a display of random dots: How many are there? Were they grouped in squares or quincunxes, you could increase your estimate four or five times.

What this leads to is that in the hyperattentive state of information overload, one way to control the burden is by imposing a construction. If the distinctive features of a face or of a voice are lost in the many unrelated details, control can be restored by creating a form or meaning — let's take anger as an example. That face is angry, that voice is threatening. Hence, if the schizophrenic, in a hyperattentive state, sees too much or hears too much, paranoia may be the decision in an attempt to "restore homeostasis". Another method might be to withdraw, to not participate and to ignore the input overload. Blunting of affect, even catatonia, may ensue.

What about hallucinations? Hallucinations are defined as a percept in the absence of an objective stimulus, but that only means objective stimulus to the outside observer. In the hyperattentive state, all sorts or random stimuli may come to consciousness, although they are blocked out by the normal. If I don't hear it (and of course I'm normal), then it doesn't exist. If it doesn't exist, and you hear it, it must be an auditory hallucination.

Or see it, for humans are visual creatures. Visual input serves as stimulus for a lot of behavior, including auditory. Schizophrenics talk at great length in a visual environment and are silent in the dark. The visual environment, which can serve as the trigger for a vocal response, then allows the auditory aspect of the vocal response to serve as the impetus for further talk. Klang association, a schizophrenic behavior, is an association at the level of the sound, not at the level of what the sound of the word (as a symbol) represents as a percept or means as a concept — denotes or connotes. So, said one of our patients, "When you see brown, you turn around and say what town?" Crazy talk certainly, but what about poetry, where the image and the sound are more cohesive (and therefore more coherent)? The visual trigger, like quieting a parrot by putting a cover over its cage, is demonstrated by a schizophrenic patient who came to see me in my office. A yearbook of neurology was on the shelf near the table at which we convened. Its binding indicated "1968." My patient approached the table, sat down and said (without a word from me), "Anno years pages. Anno years. Yr ears on straight. Yr nose is too." No stimulus you say, or didn't you notice it? Might one infer my patient was seeing ears and a nose, but not a face? That is a collection of parts not organized as a whole, even as she had seen a single volume, not a shelf of books.

Hallucinations are perceptual experiences in the absence of objective stimuli. Dreams are not hallucinations although they may occur, (are perceptual experiences) in the absence of verifiable stimuli. They occur in the normal (here's that word again) whereas hallucinations occur in, and in fact define, the abnormal. Only when awake is the remembered dream recognized as distinct from reality. It's true that one occurs in the waking state, the other in sleep, but what about daydreams or the less structured, less prolonged fantasies we all experience? Dreams are of interest because they are associated with vestibular-innervated rapid eye movements; they are taken as a sign of consciousness. They demonstrate flight of ideas with tangential association; they may have paranoid overtones, they occur with a waking electroencephalogram and they seem to require vestibular input. Nocturnal dreams (as distinct from daydreams) occur with rapid eye movement (REM) sleep. Sleep, in all its phases, relates to activity of the ascending reticular activating system in the broad sense. Originally described by Magoun and by colleagues,[2] the concept has been expanded to include structures outside of brainstem and nuclear components have been elucidated.

Although the sleep–wake cycle marks the extremes of activity by the ascending reticular activating system, it is evident that the extremes grade one into the other. Introspection reveals that arousal fluctuates during the day. Percepts are sharper at some times than at others. Daytime drowsiness reduces the clarity of the perceptual input which in turn reduces the level of arousal, for the nuclei described for the ascending reticular activating system receive low level input from the periphery. The feedback from higher levels (let's say from the lateral hypothalamus to brain stem nuclei) is simply feedback generated by earlier activity. So as perceptual input declines, arousal declines; as arousal declines, percept formation declines. Conversely, as arousal is heightened, percepts may change. Unnoticed aspects (attributes) may become prominent, the assembly may alter, the Gestalt may appear different, the meaning of the percept may transform. If there is a perceptual disorder in schizophrenia, one place to look for it may be not in the sensory or perceptual systems, but in the activating arousal systems on which the percepts are displayed.

A major contributor to the activating mechanism is the vestibular system by way of its nonspecific projection. Its specific projection relates to the vestibulor-ocular reflexes and to the multimodal projections to the cortex. It has prominent interactions at each level of representation with the visual system. The interaction contributes to, and conditions, visual perception. The perceptual abnormality in schizophrenia, as best I can tell, is not an abnormality of the visual aspects of vision, but of something analogous to a refractive aspect of vision: A normal scene viewed through a distorting lens. The scene appears tipped or wavy, aspects that are attributable to an altered vestibular system. The abnormality, presumably occurring in the multimodal cortex, is not of visual input, but of vestibular input — not only too much (or too little), but more importantly, out of balance.

Chapter 6

HALLUCINATIONS

Hallucinations are a cardinal positive symptom of schizophrenia which deserve careful study in the hope it will give information about the pathophysiology of the disorder. Defined as a sense perception not founded on observable reality, hallucinations are internally generated; the site of generation — where in the brain — is a matter of interest. The problem that arises relates to the word "observable". Presumably, that refers to an outside observer; whether external reality is observable tells as much about the observer as it does about the patient. If, as predicated, the positive symptoms of schizophrenia are an expression of a hyperalert awareness, the patient may see or hear things present in reality not visible or audible to the observer. They may be misconstrued by the patient because too much stands out. Distinctive features are not recognized as such, but if misconstrued, the hallucination is really an illusion — a false interpretation of a real sensory image, and not an internally generated image, except insofar as ultimately, every percept is internally generated. So, the first problem is to determine whether the alleged hallucination relates to an event in the real world (see Appendix).

If it does not, there are two additional problems to clarify, if possible: (1) Where in the nervous system is the hallucination generated? (2) How closely does the generated information correspond to the reported hallucination? To start with the second, the contention is that the nervous system always operates on sensory input even if that input is internally generated. Perception, as we have seen, depends not only on the external input, but also on memory, previous percepts, emotional state, level of alertness, attention and other factors. This operation is evident every day and in the normal, the evidence is every where: You drive along a residential street on a breezy autumn day and a small gust blows a mass of leaves or a piece of newspaper between two cars parked along the street Automatically, you step on the brake as you think, "a dog" or even worse, "a child". That is not what you saw, but the nervous system knows that movement means life and life means an animal or even a human.

What the schizophrenic reports must be interpreted skeptically. Assuming there is nothing in the external environment to have precipitated the "hallucination" does the report really represent it? We usually ask a patient, as I have written elsewhere, "Are you hearing voices?" when we should ask "What are you hearing?" We follow up with the question "What are the voices saying?" and are told something like "Bad things." That is not an answer to the question, so we pose it again. This time the reply might be, "They're calling me names." Still not an answer to the question. Why not? Perhaps because the voices are not saying well-articulated words; they are just noise or sounds accompanied by a limbic-generated feeling tone construed by the patient, operated on, to be "bad things". It has always seemed to me that many so-called hallucinations in toxic states, seizures or drug-induced states as well as in schizophrenia are really illusions related to a real, if unobserved, environmental stimulus. For true, internally generated hallucinations, I have never been convinced the reported hallucination represents a well formed, internally generated percept; rather it is a combination of an internally generated sensory event (visual, auditory, somatosensory) and a limbic discharge, endowing the sensory component with an affective cloak. Sound, plus the negative limbic aspect, becomes names and being called names is bad. Paresthesias become bugs and bugs are frightening. Even in the normal, this occurs: You sit on a hillside on a sunny summer day, your bare arm behind you, supporting you as you lean back. A gentle breeze blows a blade of grass across the hairs of your forearm. "A bug" you think, and usually strike at it. You can visualize that bug — a thin-waisted ant perhaps. You don't think, "a moving somatosensory stimulus". You operate on it, turn it into a bug. A hallucination for your companion who did not see the blade of grass.

Where the hallucination is generated in the nervous system may be a question without an answer. We can look to normals in whom nocturnal dreams are usually generated without external stimuli — that is stimuli from the environment whether internal — a full bladder — or external — a noise. In many ways, dreams are similar to the hallucinations of the schizophrenic: disjointed, tangential with flight of ideas. "In our sleep, we all intermittently experience insanity."[161] "In dreaming sleep, hallucinations, perceptual distortions, bizarre thinking and temporary delusions are ultimately mixed with more normal thought and perceptual processes."[162] Hughlings Jackson and Wilhelm Wundt reflected on the similarities of psychosis and of dreaming we are told. But dreams, like most non-schizophrenic hallucinations, are largely visual. There may be an auditory component, but the major aspect of the dream is visual although the congenitally blind have vivid dreams but see nothing.[161] So, it is too with hypnagogic or hypnopompic hallucinosis[163] and with the hallucinations of toxic states or delirium.

The site of initiation of the schizophrenic hallucination — internal or external — can perhaps be explored by an examination of dreaming, insofar as dreams represent an analog of hallucinations. For the most part, dreams occur during paradoxical sleep. The brain is active, the body is not. The electrographic brain is aroused, the body is behaviorally asleep. The usual source of input to the activating system is reduced, for sensory activity is markedly diminished; vision occluded, audition lessened, somatic sensation limited and pain — the major contributor to the arousal system — usually absent. What then stimulates the arousal mechanism to produce a desynchronized electroencephalogram? Only the eyes are moving, indicating an active vestibular system, and vestibular input is alleged to be the most important contributor to the reticular activating system after pain. Whether the vestibular input and eye movements generate dreams (which less frequently may occur in the absence of REM) or the eye movements are caused by the visual panorama of the dream cannot be determined, but in either case, the vestibular system (both its specific contribution to eye movements and its nonspecific contribution to arousal) is active during the hallucinatory dream. This argues for an internal genesis, although some dreams (urinating endlessly in the presence of a full bladder) are precipitated by external (that is bodily rather than primary brain) events. So, the postulate is that the schizophrenic hallucination is often externally stimulated, but may be internally generated and depends on an active or overactive vestibular system. The unresolved question is: Why is the schizophrenic hallucination primarily auditory and the hallucinatory dream primarily visual?

Daydreams are more difficult to comment about. They may have a visual component, but they usually have a coherent primary psychic scenario. Daydreaming, like night dreaming, is associated with a roughly 90-minute cycle. Penfield was able to produce dreams by stimulating the superior middle and inferior temporal gyri (if one is to judge from the diagrams) on either side. He distinguishes dreams from the "dreamy state" of Hughlings Jackson. These are illusions in which the patient may become aware of a sudden difference of his interpretation of the environment. This altered perception may take the form of *déjà vu*, or of *jamais vu*. The dream induced by cerebral stimulation is a hallucination with no relation to the real environment.

Just as electrical stimulation of the cortex can produce hallucinations, so can the stimulation of nerve cells by a seizure focus. The modality and the complexity is determined by the site of the epileptogenic focus. Visual, auditory, olfactory, somatic and gustatory hallucinations occur, representing the

five classical senses, but other senses or sensations may appear. Vertigo, dizziness, levitation, floating, flying, anxiety, familiarity, unfamiliarity and other
hallucinatory or illusory states occur. The hallucination may be elementary —
a flash of light, a sound, a smell, a taste or a somatic sensation (but usually
not pain) — or it may be complex — a visual panorama with or without
movement, a piece of music or a voice, a complex somatosensory feeling. This
may be a prelude to a more outspoken motor convulsion, or it may constitute the entire seizure. Usually if the patient recollects the event, it is
recognized as a hallucination.

Hallucinations occur as well in the non-demented individual deprived of
sensory input. To be included in this category, I believe, the sensory loss
should be peripheral. Loss of ocular visual input may be accompanied by
vivid visual scenes — the so-called Charles Bonnet syndrome, named after
the man who described it in his grandfather in 1760 — or loss of auditory
peripheral input with associated hallucinatory occurrence of noise or of
sounds. One wonders about Beethoven and the striving, inexpressible quality of the Grosse Fugue and other of the late quartets. My speculation is that
this phenomenon is created at the next waystation from the periphery, just
the way the Bechterew compensation phenomenon adjusts for the loss of
labyrinthine input.

Other normal hallucinatory events occur. Hypnagogic hallucinosis
or hypnopompic hallucinosis occurs in the normal individual at the transition
from sleep to wake or from wake to sleep respectively. More likely to occur in
the narcoleptic, these hallucinations are usually visual, but may be auditory or
tactile. They are usually without associated affect, but can be pleasant or
frightening and be hard to distinguish from reality. They are brief and recognized as not real upon waking. In the narcoleptic, they may be auditory — as
if the teacher called on you in class. In this scenario, the hallucinating
narcoleptic stands up in response to being called, only to be told to please
sit down.

In a number of dementing disorders, hallucinations may occur. Part of
the problem here is to dissociate the effect of medication — L-DOPA in
the Parkinsonian for example, or memantine in patients with Lewy body
dementia[164,165] — from the disorder itself. However, in some patients with
Lewy body dementia, visual hallucinations may appear in advance of conspicuous dementia, though this is difficult to calibrate because dementia is a
criterion of diagnosis.[166] Statements like "At the outset of the disease, patients
with DLB" (Lewy body dementia) "have presented primarily *visual hallucination*,"[167] are unclear as to whether this means visual hallucinations before
dementia, visual hallucinations with early dementia, or following the onset of

dementia, the type of hallucination is primarily (that is, usually) visual. The visual hallucinations are associated with hypometabolism on Positron Emission Tomography scan in the temporoparietal occipital association areas and the medial and lateral occipital lobes.[167] Decreased perfusion in primary and secondary visual cortex has been shown with Single Photon Emission Computed Tomography (SPECT) and Lewy body density is increased in the anterior and the inferior temporal lobe.[166] Visual hallucinations are described as complex and fully formed although all that is known is what the patient reports seeing: people, animals, objects. In contrast, auditory hallucinations, which occurred in 13% of those with visual hallucinations, are elementary: banging, knocking, sizzling a doorbell, footsteps and unintelligible voices.[168] This is of great interest with respect to the auditory hallucinations of schizophrenia. We are told the hallucinations come early in the disease — before conspicuous dementia. It is not that these patients with Lewy body dementia cannot operate on the sensation because of dementia; rather, the hallucination appears without affective accompaniment. Banging, knocking and sizzling are relatively neutral sounds and the visual hallucinations in these patients are often without affect. So it is interesting that "Amygdala-predominant pathology is...present at 60% of the frequency of a DLB (dementia with Lewy body) consensus/Braak stage conforming pattern".[169] Visual hallucinations may or may not be lateralized, may be recognized as not real and are usually without associated affect of fright or pleasure. REM sleep behavior disorder (RBD), often a harbinger of Parkinsonism, is thought to be an acting out of dreams — a hallucinatory state that expresses itself.[170] Visual hallucinations without RBD also occur in postencephalitic Parkinsonism[49] with reports of, "A man with a knife", "Flowers", and "A big black dog", which brings us back to dreams. Are dreams and hallucinations the same? "All dream images seem real at the time."[171] The discrimination between dreams and reality can be made only after waking.

Although dreams occur during REM sleep, REM sleep is not required for dreaming. Dreams also occur in NREM sleep. REM dreams tend to be narrative, NREM more basic: terrors, bugs, levitation. In RBD, the usual muscle atonia is separated from the REM stage of sleep. In the same way, dreaming can be dissociated from REM sleep.[172] "...Dreaming and REM sleep are dissociable states, controlled by distinct, though interactive, mechanisms. Dreaming turns out to be generated by the forebrain instinctual–motivational circuitry",[173] although this is not a necessary conclusion from the observation that "...dreaming stops completely when certain fibers deep in the frontal lobe have been severed". It's an old story. Function loss consequent upon a lesion does not mean that the function resides at the site of the lesion. It may not reside anywhere. It may be the product of a distributed process. The fact that "The lesion is the same as the damage that was deliberately produced in prefrontal leukotomy" is of interest, but may refer to the type of "hallucination" — visual in dreaming, auditory in schizophrenia — rather than the process that generates a false perception. Not all schizophrenics ceased hallucinating following a leucotomy. Did they stop dreaming?

Hobson, who believes that dreaming is initiated in the brain stem, rebuts the importance of a frontal fiber system. In "Freud returns? Like a bad dream", he writes, "...activating the parts of the limbic system that produces anxiety, anger and elation, shapes dreams."[174] Meanwhile, I believe activating parts of the limbic system shapes hallucinations in the schizophrenic. Ponto-geniculate-occipital waves have been correlated with dreaming, although until recently, ponto-geniculate-occipital waves have not been demonstrated in humans and dreaming has not been demonstrated in animals.[175] "...Intra-brain stem and brain stem–thalamic circuits generate the ponto-geniculate-occipital (PGO) waves that are the physiologic correlate of the internal activation of the brain during REM sleep, 'the stuff that dreams are made of'".[146] Despite the restricted projection territory suggested by the name, ponto-geniculate-occipital waves are widespread in the thalamus and the cortex beyond the geniculate and the visual cortex, and the PGO generation may be driven from the spinal cord, the brain stem, the hypothalamus and the cerebral cortex. PGO waves may appear half a minute before the electrically determined REM (by EEG and EMG), occur during REM sleep in bursts of 3–10 waves usually correlated with eye movements and can be recorded in the nuclei of the extraocular muscles. They require input to the lateral geniculate body from the medial and descending vestibular nuclei[176] to sustain the clusters of PGO waves,[177] which may be associated with dreaming, but single PGO waves persist following the destruction of the medial and descending vestibular nuclei. PGO waves are not recorded during sleep from the human scalp. Still, the brain stem origin of dreams, whether or not by PGO waves, is generally accepted. "Chaotic phasic signals arising in the pontine brain stem constantly impinge upon, and sometimes disrupt, ongoing processes in the sensory and motor centers of the cortex and subcortex of the forebrain and in emotion centers of the limbic forebrain. These signals are thought to lead directly to the visual and motor hallucinations, emotional intensification, and the distinctly bizarre cognition that characterizes dream mentation."[178]

How much of this can be verified by imaging? With respect to PGO waves or other brain stem initiators, one study showed an increase of regional cerebral (sic) blood flow in the pontine tegmentum.[179] In addition, flow was increased in the left thalamus (all 30 subjects were right handed), both amygdaloid complexes, the anterior cingulate cortex and the right parietal operculum. Often results are conflicting. Another study[180] reports the activation of the occipital cortex with the deactivation of the frontal cortex during REM. A third confirms deactivation of the inferior and middle frontal cortex but also of the inferior parietal cortex.[181] Another indicates activation of extrastriate visual cortices with attenuation of activity in the primary visual cortex,[182] as well as frontal association area reduction on the Positron Emission Tomography (PET) scan. Relative metabolism during REM sleep is increased in the hippocampus, the amygdala, the ventral striatum, the basal ganglia, the supplementary motor area,[183] the subgenual, the pregenual and anterior cingulate cortex, the medial prefrontal and the primary sensory motor cortex.[184] These studies suggest that schizophrenic hallucinations are not REM intrusions into wakefulness. In their original report of "Regularly occurring periods of eye motility and concomitant phenomena during sleep",[185] Azerinsky and Kleitman noted that eye movements and "probably dreaming" are related. We now know that dreaming occurs in REM sleep but does not require eye movements. What it does require, however, is participation by thalamocortical specific and nonspecific loops, as judged from the 40-Hz oscillation that characterizes the human dream state. This suggestion has such wide implication, it will be quoted at length:

> In addition to the finding that the electrical activity during waking and oneiric states is quite similar, a second significant finding was that during the dreaming state, 40-Hz oscillations are not reset by sensory input, although evoked potential responses indicate that the thalamoneocortical system is similarly accessible to sensory input in both states. This we consider the central difference between dreaming and wakefulness. It indicates that we do not perceive the external world during REM sleep because the intrinsic activity of the nervous system does not place sensory input in the context of the functional state being generated by the brain at that time. We may consider the dreaming condition a state of hyperattentiveness in which sensory input cannot address the machinery that generates conscious experience.

The hyperattentiveness recalls the notion that this also functions in schizophrenia.

> Beyond this we theorize that a similar mechanism may also be found in conditions where hallucinations are evoked and while 'daydreaming' where the immediate happenings of the external world may be ignored. Relating to the morphophysiological basis for this scanning property, a very attractive

hypothesis could be that the nonspecific thalamic system — in particular, the intralaminar complex — may be an important part of this process. Indeed, the intralaminar complex represents a cellular mass that projects to the most superficial layers of all cortical areas to include primary sensory cortices in a spatially continuous manner. The cells in this group may also have the necessary interconnectivity to sustain a propagation wave within the nucleus, which could result in the 40-Hz phase shift observed at the cortical level. This possibility is particularly attractive given that the damage of the intralaminar system results in lethargy, coma and that the electrophysiological properties of single neurons, especially during REM sleep, firing with a 30 to 40-Hz periodicity as in keeping with the macroscopic magnetic recordings observed in this study."[186]

Schizophrenic hallucinations are different. They are usually auditory, not visual as in these other states. Why should that be? Once again, there are two possibilities: One is that they are generated by external stimuli brought to the fore by the hyperattentive state; the second is that they are generated internally. If externally generated by the overalertness, why should they be auditory? It may be the schizophrenic hears too much for example; we know that to be true from their responses to environmental sounds such as the overhead airplane, but we also know them to be particularly attentive to the visual environment. This is evident not only from their behavior — the scraps of visual input that get incorporated into spontaneous speech — but also from the dark–light ratio of talk. If the hallucinations are a response to external stimuli, we should have expected visual hallucinations — so prominent in other disorders as well as in normals — rather than auditory, to occur.

If internally produced where do the hallucinations arise? Any decision is speculative for wherever in the auditory pathways they begin, they presumably reach the auditory cortex in the temporal lobe. They could be produced in the cortex, as happens with electrical stimulation at surgery or with a seizure disorder but they could also be initiated as far downstream as the organ of Corti. If the hallucinations arise internally, how are the auditory hallucinations and the postulated hyperactive vestibular system related? Does the intriguing observation of anastomosis between the vestibular nerve and the auditory system play a role? This has been variously considered as:

(1) a connection between the saccular branch of the vestibular nerve and the cochlear nerve;
(2) cochlear nerve fibers with perikarya in the saccular division of the vestibular ganglion;
(3) vestibular receptor fibers joining the cochlear nerve;

(4) an aberrant cochlear bundle;
(5) primary afferent cochlear fibers;
(6) afferent vestibular fibers supplying the cochlea.[187]

However viewed, it could account for vestibular hyperactivity conducting auditory impulses to awareness–auditory impulses that can remain unstructured but be interpreted as words. PET scans of five schizophrenics taken during hallucinations suggest that the origin is downstream from the temporal cortex. The scans also showed the activation of the striatum and the thalamus as well as of the hippocampus, the orbital cortex, the parahippocampal region and the cingulate cortex.[188,189] Magnetic resonance studies have shown that auditory hallucinations correlate with the reduced size of the superior temporal gyrus,[94] but that gyrus is also concerned with vestibular function. At least two problems are raised by observations of this sort. The first is the conflation of structure and function. A non-functional imaging study shows only morphology. The relationship between morphology and positive pathological function is only speculative at best. Why, for example, should auditory hallucinations arise from a temporal gyrus that is reduced in size? Reduction in size may mean a decreased number of nerve cells, but it more likely indicates a reduced neuropil. Why should reduced fiber connections (or a decreased cell population) be associated with auditory hallucinations? The hallucination is a positive event, something happening. It must be associated with a neuronal discharge. If reduced size of the superior temporal gyrus implies tissue loss — a negative phenomenon — then the auditory hallucination must be a release phenomenon generated somewhere else. In hallucinations of "organic" disease, diencephalic lesions correlate with auditory hallucinations.[190] The hypometabolism of Wernicke's and associated auditory areas support the notion that the hallucinations arise elsewhere.[191] But the hallucination is episodic, like a seizure, so it is not a release analogous to a movement disorder. We need a mechanism to account for the intermittent nature of the hallucination.

The second problem relates to functional imaging, which is only of value when the abnormality being evaluated takes place. Otherwise, functional imaging is no different from morphologic imaging. Therefore hallucinations must be assessed by a dynamic technique only as they occur. One study attributes failure to associate self-produced speech with one's self to abnormal laterality of the supplementary motor area activity, allowing inner speech to be generated without attribution and therefore be experienced as an auditory hallucination.[192] Two problems come to mind with this study as well. The first relates to "inner speech" — a Jacksonian term. Whatever it is, it is more likely language than it is speech, despite the claim of disordered monitoring of inner speech which is described as "thinking in words" as demonstrated by the reduced activation of left middle temporal gyrus and the rostral supplementary motor area.[193] It is not prearticulatory articulation; it is the formulation of a concept in an inarticulate mode. Do I know what I am going to say before I say it? Only in a most general way; the words present themselves at the moment of production. I do not hear them in my mind before I utter them, and then attribute them to an outside source.

The second problem in this formulation is that it lacks the affective component. The schizophrenic auditory hallucination is usually "bad". You might argue the words come first, then obtain an affective cloak. It seems more likely to me that the affect comes first, as Hobson suggests for dreams, then the auditory component is attached and is probably not words. This explains why it is almost impossible to get a schizophrenic to report, "What are the voices saying?" because the "voices" are not saying anything. Instead, they are making sounds attached to an unpleasant emotion or feeling. That feeling is fright or anxiety, if we must put a name on it. It is of interest that anxiety can be generated by the stimulation of the temporal lobe in a region not far from the parietal vestibular and the temporal auditory representation. Temporal lobe seizures often begin with an epigastric aura; that is where we experience anxiety, in the "pit of the stomach". "The feeling rises", the patient will tell you, "And when it reaches my head, I lose consciousness". Consider the alleged representation of the body on the cortical sensory strip. The shoulder is high on the contralateral hemisphere; the face, the lips and the tongue are near the Sylvian fissure. As stimulation proceeds onto insula, a limbic area, responses (feelings) are generated in the pharynx, larynx and abdominal viscera — the "feeling in the pit of the stomach". Other manifestations of anxiety can be generated with limbic stimulation — racing heart, elevation of blood pressure, dilated pupils. The anxiety comes first then the sense of words, but no real words, only that "they are calling me names".

One approach to the hallucination problem is to consider the possibility of a preperceptual world. There is a convincing body of evidence of processing of sensory input by the nervous system as far peripheral as the first way station, long before it comes to conscious awareness. Taking, for the moment, conscious awareness to be the ability to verbalize, to say, "I know", it is evident that preperceptual awareness occurs and that it is a late event (that is, a cortical event) in the processing chain. This preperceptual representation is actually a percept. It is poorly formed, cannot be described, is not crystallized and is largely inferred by the subject. The inference draws on memory, experience and the workings of the apperception mechanism. This is why, for most of us, a moving stimulus at ground level is a dog and not an aardvark. There is a temporary preperceptual storage area — a temporal (in the sense of time, not place, i.e. not temporal lobe) buffer zone in which the information is held prior to entering conscious awareness. So, for example, the first phoneme of a heard word must be held in storage until subsequent phonemes in the string declare it to be speech — to be processed by a linguistic analytic system — rather than another kind of sound to be processed by another kind of system. A more convincing experiment many years ago demonstrated the presence of a visual preperceptual buffer. A 5×5 matrix of single digits was tachistoscopically displayed. Immediately following display, the subject could retrieve to command any row or column of five numerals requested, implying that the entire matrix — all 25 digits — was stored. Following retrieval (or following a delay of three seconds in which no retrieval was called for), the stored array disappeared and no further retrieval was possible. Whether retrieval or whether delay extinguished the array could not be determined as the process of reciting the recovered row or column takes time. The operation of calling preperceptual information to consciousness alters, models or extinguishes the prepercept stored in the buffer.

It is as if there is a preperceptual world which is operated on to produce a percept brought to conscious awareness. To put it differently, it is as if there are two levels of "perception", two concentric worlds. The inner of the two is preperceptual and is conditioned by the outer which is apperceptual. The preperceptual is operated on by stored memories, emotions, attitudes, experiences to become apperceptual and to become verbalizable — that is, consciously aware.

That this is not farfetched is demonstrated by electrophysiologic studies. Presented with a subliminal (non-verbalizable) stimulus, the cortex responds with an evoked potential which can be recorded from the scalp. When the amplitude (strength) of the stimulus is increased, the presence of the stimulus can be verbalized. The subject is consciously aware of the stimulus and the evoked response is followed (in time) by a late event-related potential. The suggestion is that the preperceptual event correlates with the evoked potential, the storage is represented by the time delay before the appearance of the late event-related potential, when the apperceptual operation takes place and the late event-related potential correlates with the apperception and its description.

The temporal course of a stimulus from the periphery to the cortex recapitulates in time the evolution of the nervous system in space. The oldest evolutionary structures, the lowest level, are closest to the periphery. The most recently evolved are farthest away and among the last to receive a sensory impulse as it travels from the periphery, ascending serially the structures representative of evolutionary development. Thus the initial evoked potential is indicative of, and correlates with, the "preperceptual percept" at an earlier evolutionary acquisition than the late event-related potentials which indicate the "conscious awareness" produced by the action of the apperception mechanism at a higher, later evolved level. So when you jam on the brakes, you avoid the preperceptual dog which instantaneously transforms into a fluttering sheet of newsprint (in the example earlier, at the beginning of chapter).

How does all of this relate to hallucinations and their reports? The proposal is that in the presence of an overactive contribution by the vestibular system to the arousal mechanism, a hyperactive cortex is responsive to multiple irrelevant environmental stimuli which arrive in preperceptual storage. There, some are acted on by the apperception mechanism, are brought to conscious awareness, colored or structured by the contribution of apperception and are reported as the hallucination which may be a newly minted representation of the preperceptual phenomenon.

We distinguish the positive symptoms of hallucinations and paranoia one from the other. How distinct are they? Are they not but two manifestations of the same inchoate feeling — inexpressible because it is generated in the limbic system, an early cortical acquisition phylogenetically and individually. Its primacy is indicated by its five-layered cortex in contrast to the six (or more) layers of later developing and later maturing isocortex. The limbic cortex is mature before the acquisition of language, as are the feelings for which no language exists, except for metaphor.

The feeling comes first. It is overpowering, frightening. To control it, the patient gives it meaning. To control it, the patient is controlled by rays, by cosmic forces, by electrical fields, by anything just so long as it gives meaning to the inexpressible feeling. This is not very different from the way we all feel when we have a name for something. Animate or inanimate, we can control it. That is why anatomy or morphology precedes the other biological sciences. We name, classify, tabulate and group. All of this is imposed from without; it does not inhere within what is being named and classified. Is this so very different from paranoia? The botanist confronted with a multitude of new plants groups them. The hyperalert paranoid schizophrenic sees too much. To control the multitude of details, he groups by imposing meaning from without: anger, threat, external forces.

Schizophrenia, we are told, is characterized by a failure of reality testing, by impairment of perception of reality. How true is that and how do we know? In order to judge, the behavior of another is not enough, although it is all that we have. Perhaps fantasy and reality coexist (even as in the normal).

Skeptical insistence is what is needed. Instead, we bring ego and a point of view. Does the hallucinatory patient really hear voices? Do they seem real? Are they real? Are outside forces really at work? I was returning from lunch one pleasant day and joined an unknown patient walking on the grass. He was a big man I had noted several times previously, because of his hyperextended posture and the incessant athetoid sweeps of his large hands.

"Why do you moves your hands like that?" I asked.

"It's a sign of royalty". he replied.

"Yes". I said, "But why do you do it?"

"Everyone in the Royal Family does it." he answered.

"But why?" I inquired.

"It's in our blood." he said.

"But why do you keep moving your hands that way?" I asked.

"*You* know!" he said, rather impatiently. He was getting annoyed with my persistence and wanted to terminate the conversation. "It's from the medicine."

He was right on two counts. It was from the medicine and it was in the blood. But I had not listened carefully enough when he said it was in the blood. He knew at one level, perhaps did not know at another, and had imposed a story to control it. The story was of interest because there was something regal in his bearing (perhaps the extended posture resulting from the medication), although which came first, the bearing or the fantasy, is not clear. (The quotes are reconstructions).

Chapter 7

VESTIBULAR SYSTEM

The vestibular system plays a central role in my thinking about schizophrenia and a prominent role in Parkinson's disease. It is a very old system phylogenetically, having evolved from the lateral line organ of the fish.[194,195] In the human, the cortical representation myelinates earlier than the surrounding cortex. In the primate, the system is widely distributed, projecting to and receiving projections from the spinal cord, the brain stem, the thalamus, the subcortical nuclei and the cortex. Therefore, it is well positioned to have a pervasive effect on behavior. Our concern is with the diseases under discussion so an inspection of the vestibular system will be limited to areas of relevance. No attempt will be made to offer a comprehensive review of the anatomy or the physiology of the system.

Let's start with some generalities. The vestibular system is one of the major input systems. It is a sensory system, an afferent system (which, like all sensory systems, receives efferent feedback), but is never included in the five classical senses. Perhaps this is because it comes to awareness only when disturbed. It is always functioning, day and night, asleep or awake, but if it is functioning properly, we are not aware of it. Its input to central structures is widespread and diffuse, unlike the input of other sensory modalities. Lemniscal systems, projecting specific modalities, are a late phylogenetic development. Vestibular input antedated lemnisci, was distributed by reticular pathways and remains diffuse in its distribution in the brain stem, the thalamus and the cortex. Insofar as it has a lemniscus, the compact well-myelinated fibers of the medial longitudinal fasciculus connect the vestibular nuclei with the oculomotor nuclei, not with the thalamus (Fig. 10).

Of great importance in the vestibular system's functioning, is the fact that it is a tonic as well as a phasic system. It is always beating in a way that is rather different from other sensory systems. Most are silent without sensory input and even with sustained unmodified input, some stop firing. A persistent pressure on the skin, a sustained odor and we soon lose awareness of it because, unlike the vestibular system, the receptor stops firing. Vestibular

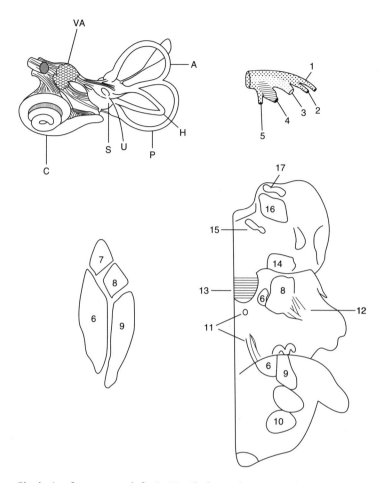

Fig. 10. Clockwise from upper left: 1: Vestibular end organ including cochlea and entire acoustic nerve; (A: Anterior canal; P: Posterior canal; H: Horizontal canal; SU: Saccule and utricle; VA: Vestibular and auditory nerve); C: Cochlea. 2: Vestibular ganglion and nerves; 3: Vestibular nuclei seen from above on right side of brain stem; 4: Three overlapping diagrams ascending right side of brain stem to show location of vestibular nuclei. 1: Anterior canal nerve; 2: Horizontal canal nerve; 3: Utricular nerve; 4: Saccular nerve; 5: Posterior canal nerve; 6: Medial vestibular nucleus; 7: Superior vestibular nucleus; 8: Lateral vestibular nucleus; 9: Descending vestibular nucleus; 10: VII nerve nucleus; 11: VI nerve and nucleus; 12: Vestibular nerve; 13: Basis pontis; 14: Superior olive; 15: VII nerve; 16: Superior vestibular nucleus; 17: Brachium conjunctivum. (Note that 7 and 16 are identical.)

nuclear adaptation does not occur.[196] The labyrinth works in conjunction with its fellow of the opposite side. When at rest, the tonic discharges of the two sides are balanced. The product or output in terms of awareness is zero, but the level of output is also being distributed to, amongst other places, the arousal system. If the level is high, for whatever reason, arousal may be increased although consciousness of the balanced output may not be. The specific aspects of the system — movement, acceleration, position — may be lacking due to the balanced output; the nonspecific aspects — hyperalertness, excessive arousal, perceptual distortion (particularly with respect to movement or rectitude of the environment), sleep disorder and even muscle tone — may become distorted.

The issue of muscle tone requires one further generalization. Muscle tone or the resistance a group of muscles offers to passive manipulation, is represented at various levels of the nervous system and is expressed as postures. When the tone — that is, the spontaneous activity — of the flexor group in a limb exceeds that of the extensor group, the posture that ensues is one of flexion. Postures are released by lesions at various levels of the neuraxis and the released posture is represented in the level of the nervous system below the lesion. So a spinal lesion releases a posture of gross flexion and the predominant posture "represented" in spinal cord is flexion. As we ascend the nervous system, postures are represented, re-represented and re-represented, becoming more refined and more delicate at each higher level. Flexion is re-represented above the red nucleus where only a segment of a given limb may be affected and again at the cortex where only flexion of a digit may be involved. The point of all of this is that the earliest instantiation of extension is at the level of the vestibular nuclei. The fastigial nucleus of the cerebellum facilitates labyrinthine tonic extension of the contralateral side of the body and alpha-rigidity collapses with a section of the VIII (vestibular) nerve.[197] When dealing with a disorder characterized by flexion, such as Parkinson's disease, we should look to regions of representation of vestibular input at higher levels or, having found the lesions first, conclude the affected nucleus represents extension.

The end organ, the membranous labyrinth, is located in the inner ear of the temporal bone adjacent to the internal auditory canal. The balance organ, it measures about one-fifth inch by one-eighth inch and is a fluid-filled (endolymph) organ surrounded by another fluid — perilymph. It is continuous with the cochlea with which the endolymph communicates by way of the ductus reuniens. The vestibular and the cochlear end organs connect with different afferent nerves — the vestibular and acoustic respectively — but both are designated as the VIII cranial nerve; an anastomosis exists between the two. The vestibular receptors consist of three semicircular canals oriented roughly to sample rotation in the three dimensions of space. Each terminates in a dilated region called the ampulla, which is a motion-sensitive cupula that responds to the inertia of the endolymph as the head moves. The canals work in pairs, one on each side of the head, and respond to rotation. If the rotation causes the crista to bend toward the ampulla of the horizontal canal, the discharge caused by its hair cells increase; if the motion of the crista is away from the lateral ampulla, the discharge in the case of the horizontal canal decreases. Deflection of the hair cell in one direction depolarizes it, in the other direction; it hyperpolarizes it, reducing transmitter release.[171] Clearly with rotation, the crista on one side of the body will be ampullopetal and on the other side, ampullofugal. For the vertical canals, ampullofugal deviation of the crista causes an increase of impulses and ampullopetal movement a decline. Motion of the cupula, generated by the inertia of the endolymph, causes a change of rate of the resting discharge for the canals are always firing tonically. At rest, the rate of discharge of a healthy canal is offset by the rate of discharge of the healthy canal of the other side, so there is no sense of motion. Motion is only sensed when the discharge rate is different on each side — whether from movement or from disease. Notice that the receptor is a three-position device, unlike some other sensory receptors which can only indicate on or off. The canal is a bidirectional indicator, as if it had a "not on" position different from "off". It is the resting level tonic discharge that creates the bidirectional character of the phasic discharge. It could be compared to an automobile which can idle in neutral, go forward or go backward. The difference is that while neutral in the analog represents the summed tonic rate of discharge and forward represents an increase from the tonic rate, reverse (which in the analogy requires increased engine output) is the result of a decrease from the tonic rate of discharge.[198]

In addition to the canals, the vestibule contains otolith organs, two on each side. The utricle responds to linear acceleration, centrifugal force and gravity. The saccule is claimed by some to respond to vibration; it can be destroyed on both sides without interfering with labyrinthine reflexes. The utricle responds to movement of the otolith, a concretious collection of crystals which is heavier than the surrounding material. It stimulates the associated hair cells to initiate a discharge. Afferent fibers originate in Scarpa's ganglion and efferent fibers project to the vestibule from many locations, including the brain stem reticular formation. Other systems — particularly vision — project to the vestibular system if not directly to the labyrinth, and the efferent labyrinthine projections can influence discharge gain.[47]

The labyrinths project to the vestibular nuclei of the brain stem where the tonic labyrinthine discharge is reflected in at least the lateral, the medial and the superior vestibular nuclei. Not all parts of each nucleus receive primary input, and input may be distinctive as well as partially common, with different primary fibers terminating in different regions.[196] The nuclear spontaneous activity persists after extirpation of the labyrinth or section of the VIII nerve and recalls the phenomenon of Bechterew's compensatory nystagmus, which may be a specific instance of a more general neurological principle also seen in recovery from spinal shock. In 1883, Bechterew reported the results of labyrinthine destruction in dogs. After one labyrinth is destroyed, recovery occurs — that is, symptoms such as nystagmus disappear, if given sufficient time. Destruction of the second labyrinth causes the recurrence of symptoms, but in the opposite direction, as if the first destroyed labyrinth were intact. This second nystagmus can be eliminated by the destruction of the vestibular nuclei on the side of the initial operation, suggesting the nuclei had compensated for the original destruction and had become spontaneously active. Destruction of the cerebellum, the cerebrum, the diencephalon, the corpora quadrigemina or the vestibular nuclei on the second side does not abolish the nystagmus produced by the second operation[69] though it is claimed that the cerebellum is involved in the mechanism responsible for compensation.[197]

There are four vestibular nuclei on each side of the brainstem. The lateral or Deiters' nucleus receives input from the semicircular canals and from the otolith organs. It projects to spinal cord by way of the lateral vestibulospinal tract to participate in postural reflexes. The descending vestibular nucleus receives input from the semicircular canals and the otolith organs and projects to the cerebellum, the reticular formation, the spinal cord and the contralateral vestibular nuclei. The medial and superior vestibular nuclei (Schwalbe and Bechterew, respectively) mainly project to the medial longitudinal fasciculus as well as to the spinal cord, having received input from the semicircular canals. The medial vestibular nucleus is mainly excitatory while the superior vestibular nucleus is largely inhibitory. The medial and descending vestibular nuclei send inhibitory impulses by vestibular activation of an inhibitory reticulospinal tract. Spinal reflexes are inhibited by dorsal root potentials in Ia afferents.[177]

The lateral vestibular nucleus is somatotopically organized. It sends ascending fibers to the reticular formation and fibers to the other vestibular nuclei, but no projections to the cerebellum. Its major efferents are to the spinal cord. However, it receives input from the cerebellum from the vermis of the anterior lobe and from the fastigial nuclei which, like the lateral vestibular nuclei, are important in spinal myotatic reflexes and muscle tone. The superior vestibular nucleus sends its long efferents rostrally by way of the medial longitudinal bundle. The afferents from the cristae accumulate in the central part of the nucleus. Those from the fastigial nuclei of both sides are arranged peripherally in the nucleus. The medial vestibular nucleus contributes from its entire area to the medial longitudinal fasciculus and from the ventrolateral part, sends fibers to the cerebellum. In addition, fibers (perhaps collaterals of rostrally directed branches) descend into the spinal cord. Fibers come from the contralateral and the homolateral fastigial nucleus, the contralateral by the hook bundle of Russel. The medial vestibular nucleus projects abundantly to the mesencephalon, receives axon collaterals from the lateral vestibular nucleus, contains internuncial cells and is therefore thought to serve an integrative function.[187,198] For example, the retina projects to the nucleus of the optic tract in the pretectum, which in turn projects to the medial vestibular nucleus. "Neurons that receive input from this nucleus" (the medial vestibular nucleus) "cannot distinguish between visual and vestibular signals."[171] The nucleus of Darkschewitsch probably contributes to visual input as it receives input from occipital cortex.[199] The descending or inferior vestibular nucleus has connections similar to those of the medial vestibular nucleus. A distinct group of fastigial-vestibular fibers can be recognized. Many afferent fibers enter the medial longitudinal fasciculus and from the caudal descending nucleus, there are cerebellar projections. Afferent fibers from the anterior vermis (homolateral and contralateral), terminate in separate locations in the nucleus and are joined by a small number of spinal afferents. Finally, it is important to note direct anatomic connections from the labyrinth to the flocculonodular lobe of the cerebellum without synapse in one of the nuclei.

The major ascending projection from the vestibular nuclei is the medial longitudinal fasciculus. For the vestibular system, this parallels the lemniscal projections of other sensory systems. However, they go to thalamus while vestibular projections to the thalamus, though plentiful, are diffuse. The medial longitudinal fasciculus correlates eye movements with head movement and by means of the vestibuloocular reflex, keeps the visual world steady — perhaps a point of interest in light of the frequent schizophrenic report of waviness and movement of the visual environment or intensification of those symptoms with bodily movements. The eyes are moved by the extraocular muscles. There are six for each eye. Eye movements are yoked; we cannot move one eye without moving the other. For any movement, lateral gaze for instance, all 12 muscles are involved; some innervated, others inhibited. This is done by the participation of the vestibular nuclei by means of the connections of the medial longitudinal bundle but also by way of the reticular formation as determined by nystagmus with labyrinthine stimulation. Nystagmus is an involuntary eye movement that accompanies smooth pursuit movements (really compensates for or returns the eyes to the starting position) and is part of the vestibuloocular reflex or represents a disturbance of the labyrinths or their connections. In all of these situations, the eyes move slowly in one direction and are returned quickly in the other. The fast phase is generated in the reticular formation.[196] Nystagmus is named by the fast component which requires an intact reticular formation, where neurons that fire synchronously with the fast component have been found.[69] The best nomenclature for nystagmus is to name it in degrees. First degree nystagmus is in the direction of gaze at the extreme of gaze: for example, first degree nystagmus to the right is when the eyes are at the extreme of right lateral gaze. Second degree nystagmus (say, to the right), when the eyes are central and third degree nystagmus is when the nystagmus is in a direction contrary to the direction of gaze, such as third degree nystagmus to the right means a gaze to the left. Lower degrees of nystagmus are subsumed, so third degree nystagmus (for example) means first and second degree are also present. First degree nystagmus bilaterally (a common form of nystagmus) is easier said than "bilateral lateral nystagmus on lateral gaze bilaterally". The presumption is the vestibular signal drives the slow phase, the brain stem reticular formation drives the fast component. The vestibulo-ocular reflex is driven by the canals and the otolith organ. The fact that nystagmus involves the vestibular apparatus and the reticular formation is important in view of the abnormality of smooth pursuit eye movements in schizophrenia.

Labyrinthine testing can be done a number of ways, but the common reproducible methods are with rotation in a Barany chair, by galvanic stimulation or by caloric testing. The caloric method is most common and consists of flushing the external ear canals with water at either a hot stimulus level of 44 degrees Centigrade which produces nystagmus (which can be timed) toward the side of irrigation or with cold water at 30 degrees Centigrade which produces nystagmus away from the stimulated canal. Corticofugal impulses participate in post-rotational and caloric nystagmus.[187]

If the medial longitudinal fasciculus is considered the analog of the lemniscal system because it is a bundle (a lemniscus), there must be another component to the specific system which traverses the thalamus, arrives at the cortex and accounts for sensations of vertigo (meaning a false sensation of movement) and of movement, including rotation. Cortical stimulation at surgery or by a seizure can produce these sensations, implying specific pathways for vestibular sensation. Cortical participation can be tested by the method of the optokinetic reflex, which we have shown can be impaired in tardive dyskinesia.[134] Optokinetic nystagmus is the kind of nystagmus that occurs while watching a moving scene. Purkinje noted it in 1825 while watching a crowd at a cavalry parade in Vienna.[69] It occurs as passengers on a train watch passing telephone poles and has also been called "railroad nystagmus".

Clearly vision plays a role as it does in what is called "miner's nystagmus" seen in those deprived of ordinary visual exposure for long periods of time.

Two mechanisms are thought to be at work independently, so there are two kinds of optokinetic nystagmus. One, in which attention is necessary, is called cortical. With decortication, the nystagmus, the slow phase of which is in the direction of movement, disappears in the ipsilateral direction if the decortication is unilateral. If, however, the cortex is spared and only the optic tract is lesioned, nystagmus persists in both directions.[200] This cortical nystagmus does not depend on the labyrinth.[132,201] The supposition is that the frontal and parietal pathways descend in the anterior limb of the internal capsule to the paramedian pontine reticular formation. Some fibers must pass to the region of the caudate, for lesions there impair the response. These pathways are thought to be the same as the pathways for pursuit and saccades. This cortical optokinetic nystagmus occurs only in foveate animals, stabilizes moving objects on the retina, is not accompanied by a sense of movement and is tested for with a rotating striped drum held before the subject in a stable environment. Nystagmus can be inhibited by looking "through the drum".

Subcortical optokinetic nystagmus, in contrast, can be elicited when both hemispheres have been removed. Fixation (and attention) is not required. All parts of the visual surroundings must move in the same direction so the subject sits inside a large striped drum and can see nothing but the stripes. This older reflex occurs in non-foveate as well as in foveate animals and produces a sense of rotation. It disappears acutely with labyrinthectomy. Fibers are alleged to leave the optic tract somewhere between the chiasm and the lateral geniculate nucleus, descend to the vestibular nuclei, the nucleus prepositus, the flocculus and the paramedian pontine reticular formation where the visual and the vestibular inputs are integrated. Optokinetic nystagmus supplements the vestibuloocular reflex (which adapts rapidly) to stabilize the visual image on the retina.[171]

Before leaving the brain stem, we should look at the nonspecific connections again, both afferent and efferent, for they are extensive, function in the arousal system (and so are pertinent to our thesis) and are concerned (among other things) with the amplitude or gain of the system. Few, if any, primary afferents go to the reticular formation, but second-order fibers to reticular formation arise in all four vestibular nuclei.[197] Efferent input to the labyrinth, as evidenced by retrograde labeling from the horizontal canal, comes from many nuclear groups in the brain stem activating system. Polysynaptic input from many sources converge on the reticular formation and form a proposed closed loop feedback system with open-loop input possible. This allows response to somatosensory input and visual input, as well as to vestibular input and provides a way to control the gain. Facilitatory and inhibitory effects of vestibular efferent neurons on vestibular afferent neurons have been demonstrated[47] and peptidergic modulators that can facilitate or attenuate responses have been found (among other places) in the periaqueductal gray and the locus coeruleus. An inhibitory tonic efferent system can allow for primary afferent increase of output if its rate of tonic discharge is decreased from above so it can be excitatory as well as inhibitory.[202] Extensive afferent projection from the medial vestibular nucleus indicates visuomotor and postural integration. Projections are traced to or from sensory and motor nuclei, including other vestibular and cochlear nuclei (auditory hallucinations?), pontine nuclei, reticular formation, oculomotor nuclei, other midbrain nuclei, thalamus and amygdala.[203]

The pathway in the brain stem to higher levels is not clear. Section of the medial longitudinal fasciculus does not interrupt cortical projection of vestibular impulses. The auditory pathways seem like a logical possibility and section of the lateral lemniscus or brachium of the inferior colliculus is alleged to interrupt conduction.[187] An intermediate pathway between the medial and the lateral lemniscus has been suggested[204] with termination in the region of the medial geniculate body. In 1961, I suggested that the termination was in the magnocellular division of the medial geniculate body,[205] and this was later confirmed by others.[206] Subsequent studies with modern techniques have substantiated this location, but only as a small part of a much larger thalamic terminus. At least ten thalamic regions excluding the nonspecific intralaminar nuclei are demonstrated to project to vestibular cortical fields in the squirrel monkey.[194] This widespread thalamic vestibular representation suggests three things: (1) Input to the thalamus was widespread and diffuse, antedating development of the lemniscal systems. (2) Cortical and subcortical representation is widespread and diffuse. (3) Vestibular input plays an import physiological and behavioral role in the economy of the organism. The lemniscal systems are a phylogenetic late development[208] as must be the circumscribed primary cortical projection areas.

Cerebellar and basal ganglia relations with the vestibular system are important. The cerebellum (Fig. 11) arises from the octavolateral area of the rhombic lip and so is closely related to the vestibular system. The entire cerebellar vermis receives vestibular input, a point of some interest in light of the imaging reports of atrophy of the cerebellar vermis in patients with schizophrenia,[209] confirmed by postmortem studies.[210] Vermis, flocculonodular lobe and fastigial nuclei have been proposed as "limbocerebellum."[211] Cerebellar size has been claimed to have predictive value of psychosocial outcome in schizophrenia.[212] The flocculonodular lobe receives primary afferents

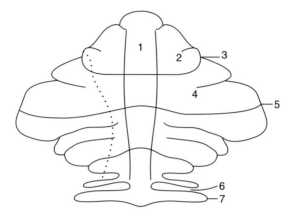

Fig. 11. Schematic representation of the opened out cerebellum displayed as if all structures were on the same plane. 1: Vermis; 2: Anterior lobe; 3: Primary fissure; 4: Posterior lobe; 5: Horizontal fissure; 6: Posterior fissure; 7: Flocculonodular lobe. Dotted line on the hemisphere demarcates intermediate zone from lateral zone. Each zone projects to its subcortical cerebellar nuclei: medial to fastigial, intermediate to globose and emboliform, lateral to dentate.

directly from the labyrinth and projects back to the end-organ.[202] It also receives input from the vestibular nuclei and projects to the lateral vestibular nucleus. Primary vestibulocerebellar fibers also project to the ventral uvula and the fastigial nucleus.[197] Labyrinthine stimulation excites the fastigial nuclei of both sides, causing tonic excitation of the labyrinthine nuclei of both sides.[197] The uvula also projects on the fastigial nuclei from the caudal part of which the hook bundle of Russell arises to project to Deiters' (lateral) nucleus of the opposite side.[78] Purkinje cells in the flocculonodular lobe inhibit cells in the medial and the lateral vestibular nuclei. There are also monosynaptic vestibular projections from the cerebellar cortex to the fastigial nucleus[78] from outside of the "vestibulocerebellum" territory. Projections to the vestibular nuclei arise in the anterior and posterior vermis and in the fastigial nuclei[197] which also project to the pontomedullary reticular formation.[213] Thus, the anterior vermis and the corresponding fastigial nuclei are allegedly important in schizophrenia.[214]

There are two pathways by which the Purkinje cell can influence the vestibular nuclei (Fig. 12): One, direct, arises in the anterior vermis and is inhibitory; the second is indirect with a synapse in the fastigial nucleus. These projections originate in the anterior and the posterior cerebellar vermis. From the fastigial nucleus, they are distributed to both sides, mainly to the lateral vestibular nucleus. Purkinje cells are inhibitory so the direct path will inhibit the lateral vestibular nucleus. The Purkinje cells of the indirect path should

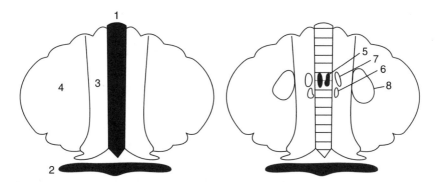

Fig. 12. Vestibulocerebellar and cerebellovestibular connections. Vermis and flocculonodular lobe receive vestibular input (left diagram). Fastigial nuclei and vermis Purkinje cells (via fastigial nuclei) along with flocculonodular lobe project back to vestibular nuclei. Schematic diagram of the cerebellum is unfolded to show anterior lobe, posterior lobe and flocculonodular lobe on a single plane. Direct projections to or from vestibular end organ or nuclei indicated in black, indirect projections, via fastigial nuclei, cross hatched 1: Vermis; 2: Flocculonodular lobe; 3: Intermediate hemisphere; 4: Lateral hemisphere; 5: Fastigial nucleus; 6: Globose nucleus; 7: Emboliform nucleus; 8: Dentate nucleus.

inhibit the fastigial projection to the Deiters' nucleus, but fastigial spinal projections increase the gain of dorsal column nuclei[215] and the lateral vestibular nucleus transmits impulses originating in the fastigial nucleus to the extensor musculature of the limbs[197] to increase extensor tone. Fastigial neurons discharge spontaneously and contribute to a reverberation with the descending vestibular nucleus. Therefore the postulate is:

1) Short and long axon Purkinje cells are inhibitory.
2) Projection of long axon Purkinje cells inhibits the vestibular nuclei.
3) Projection of short axon Purkinje cells inhibits the fastigial nucleus.
4) Labyrinthine volleys excite the fastigial nucleus which in turn creates a bilateral tonic excitatory labyrinthine background.
5) Cerebellar atrophy in schizophrenia is largely vermian in the region of vestibular afferent and efferent connections. Whether this atrophy is the cause of or the result of the fundamental process is not known.
6) If the atrophy signals dysfunction of Purkinje cells, this could indicate disinhibition of the lateral vestibular nucleus and the cerebellar fastigial nuclei.
7) This would result in heightened labyrinthine activity causing heightened ascending reticular activating system activity, producing hyperawareness with excessive response to environmental stimuli.

8) If the degenerative cerebellar process involves the fastigial nucleus as well as the vermis, decreased labyrinthine output to the ascending reticular activating system would result in apathy, disinterest and other negative symptoms.
9) The first would account for the positive symptoms of schizophrenia, the second, for the negative.
10) Fastigial, lateral vestibular nuclear output increase produces via the lateral vestibulospinal tract, the increased tone of catatonia.

One unifying hypothesis which does not require loss of Purkinje cells is this: Mossy fibers arise in brain stem nuclei. These nuclei, which include nucleus reticularis tegmenti pontis, are hyperactive so persistent stimulation of mossy fibers causes increased activity of granule cells and their parallel fibers. Parallel fibers stimulate many Purkinje cells. A single Purkinje cell can receive input from up to about 200,000 parallel fibers,[216] which have been described as the "fundamental information processing unit of the cerebellar cortex".[216] When extremely active, Purkinje cells completely suppress the vestibular nuclei directly or indirectly by way of the fastigial nuclei. This produces the negative symptoms of schizophrenia, including the lack of caloric response in catatonia and the change of muscle tone seen in waxy flexibility caused by suppression of the descending reticulospinal inhibition of alpha motor neurons which are innervated by the lateral vestibular nucleus particularly for extension. This would also account for the apathy, flat affect and the lack of participation of negative symptomatology.

The system is one of negative feedback and so should be self-stabilizing. Increased arousal produces an increase of inhibitory discharge of Purkinje cells with decreased activity of vestibular nuclei, causing decreased activity of the arousal system with damping of Purkinje cell output. However, it would only work this way as a closed system. If there were additional input from sources other than feedback, persistent inhibition could be generated until the open end of the loop changed its input, allowing the catatonic episode to subside. Mossy fiber input not only comes from primary and secondary vestibular sources, but also comes from the frontal, the parietal and the occipital cortex by way of pontocerebellar input as well as from the superior colliculus and the spinal cord, so sources for open loop input are plentiful. The corticopontocerebellar loop is also a closed loop, but it can interact with the vestibulocerebellar loop. Corticopontine input can be divided into motor and associative cortical projections. The motor outflow favors the interpeduncular and peripeduncular nuclei; association cortical projections favor rostromedial pons (prefrontal cortex), rostrolateral pons (multimodal inferior parietal cortex) dorsolateral, lateral and dorsal pons (multimodal superior temporal cortex and visual areas).[217] This motor-associative division is reflected in the pontine projections to the cerebellum. The projections from rostral pons (associative) go to the posterior cerebellar lobe and those from caudal pons (motor) project to the anterior cerebellar lobe. The posterior cerebellar lobe is thought to be involved in intellect, affect and emotion, which may explain the exuberant increase in fiber population from prefrontal regions as determined in the cerebral peduncle when human is compared to monkey.[216]

Demonstration of reduced cerebellar inhibition in schizophrenia was obtained with transcranial magnetic stimulation. Following a conditioning cerebellar stimulus, the size of a motor cortex (left) induced potential in the first dorsal interosseous was determined. Inhibition was reduced by almost 30% in schizophrenics as compared to normals in whom 50% reduction of motor cortex evoked potential occurs. This lack of inhibition correlates with the known reduction of the number of Purkinje cells per unit length of the Purkinje cell layer in schizophrenia. In this formulation, the lack of inhibition could release the vestibular nuclei and lead to a hyperattentive state but from this study, there is no way to distinguish this from involvement of cerebello-thalamic-cortical pathways.[218]

Purkinje cells project to the medial vestibular nucleus to participate in eye movements via the medial longitudinal fasiculus.[219] The vestibulocerebellar cortex receives visual input via mossy fibers from the superior colliculus and from the striate cortex which projects to the same region by way of pontine nuclei. In the frog, visual input can function at the most peripheral level of the horizontal canal.[207] Retrograde labeling (rat), following injection of lateral and medial rectus muscles revealed uptake by Purkinje cells of the flocculus and ventral paraflocculus.[220,221] Retrograde labeling following injection of flocculus-paraflocculus or nodulus-uvula (rat, gerbil), occurred in vestibular, inferior olivary, Darkschewitsch and optic tract nuclei. In addition, noradrenergic cells of the reticular formation were labeled,[222] a point of interest because nora-drenergic projections from the locus ceruleus to the anterior cerebellar vermis modify the gain of vestibospinal reflexes in the cat.[223] The meaning of cere-bellar vermis atrophy in schizophrenia is not clear but if it reflects Purkinje cell loss, as it seems to, (and Purkinje cells are known to relate to[47,203] and to inhibit[196] Dieters' and the deep nuclei of cerebellum), one might predict the loss of Purkinje cell inhibition to result in heightened or excessive arousal. Persistence of vermis serotonin 1A receptors is also claimed.[224]

Vestibular interaction with the basal ganglia is much more inferential and depends on how one defines the basal ganglia. Evidence comes in part from the clinic, in part from the physiology laboratory and in part from an anatomical

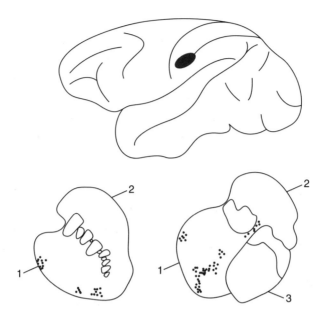

Fig. 13. Projection form cortical vestibular area in the rostroventral intraparietal sulcus of the rhesus monkey to two representative schematic levels of the striatum. 1: Putamen; 2: Caudate; 3: Globus pallidus. Stipple indicated tracer label in nerve terminals. Cortical area of injection indicated in black. Adapted from Yeterian and Pandya.

basis. The relation of decerebrate rigidity in extension to the presence of the vestibular nuclei allows for the inference that disorders such as Parkinson's disease, characterized by flexion and associated with demonstrable changes in the globus pallidus, relate to the representation of extension (a vestibular function) in the pallidum (Fig. 13). The demonstration of activation of the magnocellular medial geniculate nucleus by vestibular nerve filament stimulation[225] correlated with activation of the globus pallidus by stimulation of the magnocellular medial geniculate nucleus[226] allows the conclusion of a relationship between the vestibular nerve and the pallidum. Removal of the heads of both caudate nuclei results in a reduced influence of labyrinthine stimulation,[227] and injury of the oral part of the globus pallidus generates the conclusion that the tertiary vestibular tracts terminate in "this paleostriate center."[228] Basal ganglia nowadays is taken to mean: (1) striatum, (2) globus pallidus, (3) substantia nigra, and (4) subthalamic nucleus of Luys. Striatum is composed of two parts: a dorsal striatum of caudate and putamen and a ventral striatum, which includes the nucleus accumbens. If the substantia nigra is included in the definition, then there is good evidence of a vestibular connection[203] to the substantia nigra pars compacta which is known to project to striatum which in turn projects to the pallidum. Medial and superior vestibular nuclei are thought to project to the striatum by way of the thalamic perifascicular nucleus.[229] The ventral tegmental area, which is dopaminergic, as is the substantia nigra pars compacta, is considered as an extension of the substantia nigra pars compacta and receives input from the medial vestibular nucleus.

The role of the basal ganglia in Parkinson's disease and in schizophrenia (and therefore the role of the vestibular system) has received attention so it warrants further exploration. The internal segment of the globus pallidus is functionally related to the pars reticulata of the substantia nigra. Both use gamma-aminobutyric acid as an inhibitory transmitter. The only excitatory projection of the basal ganglia is the glutaminergic projection from the sub-thalamic nucleus of Luys to the substantia nigra and to both segments of the globus pallidus. Tonic activity of the striatum is controlled by local inhibitory neurons. Input comes from intralaminar thalamic nuclei, cortex (glutaminergic) mesencephalon (dopaminergic) and raphé nuclei (serotonergic). Output comes from the internal segment of the globus pallidus and the pars reticulata of the substantia nigra, both of which are tonically active. There are two output pathways. A direct pathway allows for phasic activation from the striatum to suppress the tonically active pallidum which inhibits the thalamus and brain stem nuclei. This allows for the activation of the thalamus and the cortex. An indirect pathway when phasically active, inhibits the thalamus. The direct pathway, by suppressing the globus pallidus, produces positive feedback and facilitates movement; the indirect pathway by negative feedback inhibits the thalamus and inhibits movement. In Parkinson's disease, decreased DOPA from the pars compacta of the substantia nigra increases the activity of the indirect path and decreases the activity of the direct path by means of the D_1 and D_2 receptors respectively. This increases the activity of the internal segment of the pallidum to increase inhibition of the thalamus and the mesencephalic tegmental neurons producing hypokinesis.

The basal ganglia are also responsible for saccadic eye movements. From frontal and supplementary eye fields, projections go to the caudate, to the substantia nigra pars reticulata, to the superior colliculus and to the frontal eye fields. Because the basal ganglia are involved in both extrapyramidal and psychiatric disorders, schizophrenia might be viewed as "Parkinson disease of thought". By this analogy, schizophrenic symptoms would arise from disordered modulation of prefrontal circuits",[230] although it is not clear what is meant by "modulation" (neuromodulators).

All of this — the vestibular bidirectional relationship with the medial longitudinal fasciculus, the thalamus, the basal ganglia — can be considered as a type of specific, even if non-lemniscal, projection; but there are rich, nonspecific projections to the arousal system in which the vestibular input plays an important role. Extensive connections exist between the medial vestibular nucleus and the sleep-arousal system as well as with the orexin system, and the circadian system. Connections exist with the locus coeruleus, the pedunculo-pontine nuclei, the raphé nuclei, the reticular formation nuclei, and other pontine nuclei as well as the ventral tegmental area, the substantia nigra and the hypothalamus.[203] This suggests a powerful role in the arousal system and a potential role in any disorder in which the arousal system is disrupted. "Vestibular stimuli cause more arousal reactions than any other sensory stimuli, except for pain... Vestibular stimuli tend to produce nonspecific responses in all cortical areas... Specific responses have a constant and short latency... nonspecific responses have a variable long latency... and often persists for a long time after the end of the stimulus. Most neuronal responses to vestibular stimuli... are of this nonspecific type."[195] The speculation is that feedback from the reticular formation by the vestibular efferents can amplify or reduce (depending on whether positive or negative feedback) the vestibular afferent output, causing heightened arousal, increased feedback, oscillation. In the case of heightened arousal, it can amplify or reduce noise and perceptual intrusions or in the case of diminished feedback, torpor, stupor, apathy and disinterest.

The vestibular cortical field is widespread and may not constitute a primary projection area in the sense that other sensory symptoms have primary then secondary and farther fields of elaboration. Normal vestibular function does not create a percept; it contributes to percepts formed by input from other modalities — particularly vision with which the vestibular system has important interaction, perhaps by way of projection from the medial vestibular nucleus to the intergeniculate leaflet[231] or its homolog. In our experiments in cats (in which Larry Murphy took an important part), widespread cortical response appeared with electrical stimulation of the ampulla of the horizontal canal. Responses were of maximal amplitude in the region of the descending anterior suprasylvian gyrus but extended widely in all directions. At the time, I considered all responses to be the analog of a lemniscal response by way of the thalamus to a primary projection area. I attributed the widespread distribution to the fact that the animals, which had been spinal-ized and treated with local anesthetic, were awake, allowing the full territory of primary projection to be displayed. Now, in retrospect, I wonder if the response was not a display of a vestibular component of the arousal system. Perhaps the reason that "vestibular cortex" is so elusive is because it does not have a primary projection area; it is not a modality like other sensory modalities. It cannot work alone (like, say vision), but it requires a combination of exteroceptors, proprioceptors, and even interoceptors (we know vestibular activity plays a role in autonomic function) on which to operate. It even interacts with the motor cortex where 50% of the cells (cat) respond to vestibular stimuli.[195] Widespread distribution of response occurs in humans. Functional Magnetic Resonance Imaging was performed during caloric stimulation (both sides individually). Activation maps with right hemisphere dominance showed response in the temporoparietal junction, the posterior and anterior insulae, pre- and post-central gyrus, areas in parietal lobe, the ventrolateral occipital lobe and the inferior frontal gyrus.[232] Electrical stimulation at surgery produced vestibular symptoms from 44 sites in 28 patients. Vestibular areas were found in the temporal, the parietal, the frontal, the occipital and the insula cortex with a particularly effective region in the perisylvian area.[233] The most effective zone in the cat is the anterior suprasylvian gyrus, which is often spoken of as the composite gyrus because it is multimodal. It is responsive to somatosensory and auditory input, as well as to vestibular input. Multisensory convergence also occurs in the Macaque (Fig. 14), where it is located in the posterior superior temporal plane. Somatosensory and auditory responses can be recorded here and projections to visual areas have been shown. These polysensory areas receive thalamic input from nuclei known to mediate vestibular activity including the magnocellular medial geniculate body and the ventral posterior inferior nucleus which are recognized as multisensory nuclei (Fig. 15).[234,235] Even in the vestibular nuclei of the brain stem, convergence of modalities (vestibular and deep somatic) has been found.[195] The uncertainties regarding the vestibular thalamus of the past are yielding to new techniques. The result is a reassessment of vestibular cortex and perhaps a reassessment of the role of the vestibular system as it relates to

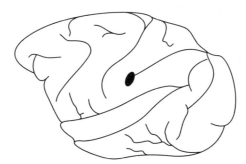

Fig. 14. Primary cortical vestibular area of rhesus monkey located at the lateral end of the intraparietal sulcus. Evoked responses were obtained under barbiturate anesthesia following stimulation of the contralateral vestibular nerve.

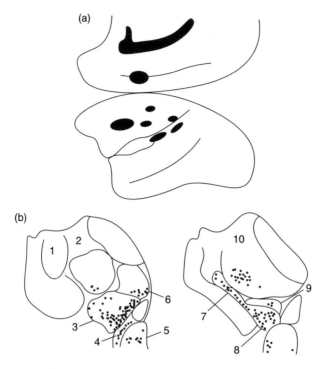

Fig. 15. (A) Cortical areas projecting to brain stem ventricular complex of squirrel monkey (from Akbarian *et al.*[236]). Medial aspect of hemisphere above. Insula and cingulate sulcus opened. Widespread areas of cortex project to vestibular nuclei. (B) Two levels of schematic view of squirrel monkey thalamus following retrograde tracer injection into insula. Stipple indicates labelled cells. Individual nuclei identified by number. 1: Dorsomedial; 2: Oromedial pulvinar; 3: Posterior nucleus; 4: Magnocellular medial geniculate body; 5: Parvocellular medial geniculate body; 6: Ventroposterior nucleus; 7: Nucleus limitans; 8: Suprageniculate body; 9: Posterior nucleus; 10: Medial posterior nucleus.

the other senses. Using the retrograde tracer technique in the squirrel monkey,[194] more than ten thalamic nuclei have been identified following injection at five cortical sites known to be areas of vestibular representation: ventral lateral, ventral posterior group (oral, superior, lateral, medial, posterior and inferior nuclei) posterior, suprageniculate, limitans, magnocellular medial geniculate, pulvinar (oral and medial), paracentralis, central lateral, central medial, and centrum medianum (Fig. 15B). From this array, six or perhaps seven were chosen on the basis of two criteria: (1) structures which receive terminals from afferent vestibulothalamic fibers, and (2) thalamic nerve cells which respond to vestibular stimulation. Candidates for vestibular function are central lateral, central posterior oralis, ventral posterior superior, ventral posterior inferior, ventral posterior lateral, ventral posterior posterior, and perhaps magnocellular medial geniculate if confirmed by single unit recordings during vestibular stimulation. In the rat,[229] vestibular input is listed for nine thalamic nuclei (ventral lateral, ventral posterolateral, lateral dorsal, central lateral, perifascicular, ventral basal complex, suprageniculate, magnocellular medial geniculate, and ventral nucleus of the medial geniculate) which project respectively to the motor cortex, area 3a, area 7 limbic and visual systems, frontal eye field area 7, striatum, insula cortex areas 2 and 7, insula frontal eye fields and area 7, auditory and insula cortex, auditory cortex. A separate study finds connections between the vestibular nuclear complex of the squirrel monkey and the parietoinsulovestibular cortex, area 7 anterior, vestibular fields of area 3a, temporal cortex bordering the insula, premotor area 6a and anterior cingulate cortex 6c and 23c.[236] This widespread distribution can be construed as indicating multiple vestibular areas but it seems more likely that vestibular input interacts with many other inputs at cortical levels, just as it does at lower levels. Extensive overlap has been shown even in the primary sensory cortex. Primary projection areas are increasingly recognized to be multimodal, although "modal" is not the correct term for vestibular input as it is not a sensory mode in the strict sense. Its non-lemniscal, multithalamic, widespread cortical distribution suggests interaction and conditioning of the more classical sensory modalities with non-modality specific conditioning of perception just as non-modality limbic input determines the affect of a percept. This "specific"contribution of the vestibular system plays a role partway between the activating system (to which it contributes) and the classical sensory systems.

So, for a tiny organ of balance in the inner ear, there is a widespread distribution and an enormous control. Projections go to the brain stem to powerfully influence arousal and to control eye movements. Output goes to the thalamus and to the cortex to contribute to perception by the classic modalities. Basal ganglia receive input that modulates posture and motor control. Motor control is generated by spinal cord that receives direct and indirect vestibular impulses. Finally, the cerebellum obtains vestibular information and, like all of the other systems, returns information to the vestibular system. We often think of the various afferent and efferent systems as linear and as operating in series. They are really better thought of as a group of interconnected concentric loops that operate in parallel. Each level feeds back on itself as well as contributing to higher and lower levels. In that way, the vestibular system has widespread effect on all behavior, conscious and unconscious. When disturbed, it can manifest itself acutely (vertigo with nausea) or can indicate its abnormality in a chronic disturbance such as Parkinson's disease or schizophrenia.

Chapter 8

TEMPORAL LOBE EPILEPSY

Suppose one were to look at it from the other side. Instead of starting where the vestibular system begins, in the labyrinth or the vestibular nuclei, suppose one were to start where the vestibular system ends. The cortical termination is not exactly known in man, but it is in the general vicinity of the superior temporal gyrus, in its posterior extent as well as in the adjacent inferior parietal lobe. It is near the primary acoustic cortex, just as you would expect, since the vestibular system starts adjacent to the auditory receptors in the cochlea, travels (as best we know) in close company with the auditory projections, perhaps finds a thalamic waystation adjacent to the auditory and in the cat, at least, ends in a cortical region that serves auditory and somatosensory input — the so-called composite gyrus. It should be no surprise that it arrives at a multimodal area, for vibration, which is allegedly monitored by the saccule, like low tones (on the organ for example), can be felt by somatosensory input as well as heard.

The relation of the temporal cortex to the vestibular system is indicated by the occurrence of vertigo with vestibular cortical stimulation in a human, awake at surgery. Some instances of temporal lobe epilepsy begin with a vertiginous aura, while others include getting up (if sitting or lying) and turning around or walking around in a small circle, reminiscent of an animal in which one labyrinth has been destroyed; the remaining active labyrinth generates the circling behavior. So in the case of temporal lobe epilepsy, the overactive, unbalanced vestibular cortex of the epileptic side results in circling. In extreme cases, it is spoken of as the "whirling dervish syndrome".

Penfield, who has had extensive experience stimulating the brain of the awake human, locates vestibular symptoms in the region adjacent to auditory projections.[237] In one case, a sense of rocking was produced by stimulation posterior to the primary auditory projection area. In a diagram, Penfield locates the vestibular field as a band just inferior to the auditory area and in a second diagram, shows the location of the labyrinthine responses from 108 temporal explorations in the same area. Symptoms experienced were "dizziness all over", "things turning around, whirling", "dizziness", "moving around", "swinging, spinning".

Temporal lobe epilepsy has an interesting aspect that is usually not commented on. As I have seen it, the symptomatology is partially dependent on the age of onset or, more accurately, on the age of acquisition of the lesion that ultimately causes the symptoms of epilepsy and its consequence. If acquired in adult life after the cortex has matured, it produces a circumscribed symptom complex representative of the neuronal discharge. The behavior pattern may be complex, the discharge incomplete, that is, not proceeding to a tonic-clonic motor seizure with complete loss of consciousness. It is spoken of as a partial complex seizure and the epileptic performance is often quite complex, but between seizures, behavior is normal. For example, I had one patient who entered a hospital nursing school at almost 20 years of age. Rooms with double-decker bunk beds were assigned, and my patient was paired with a very overweight young woman as a roommate. They flipped a coin for bed choice and having won, my patient chose the lower bunk. On the first night, undoubtedly a restless one, the upper spring, mattress and the upper occupant descended upon my patient, causing a fracture of the thin right temporal squama. It was not long before she developed a stereotyped seizure disorder. Each spell lasted less than half a minute and consisted of her rising (if she were sitting or lying), lifting her flexed left forearm to chest level, turning slightly to the left and looking at her wristwatch, whether or not she was wearing a watch. On recovery, she had no recollection of the event. Between seizures — which responded well to medication — she performed normally, completed school satisfactorily and pursued her career as a competent nurse.

At the other extreme is the temporal lobe seizure disorder that begins in very early life, before the nervous system is mature. It is as if the epileptic focus determined the subsequent maturation of the temporal cortex, much like the way the organizer of Spemann determines the development of the rest of the organism,[238] or the way the notochord determines the development of the overlying neural tube. Destroy a part of the notochord and a part of the ultimate spinal cord, for example, will not develop. Obviously, this is an early life event. Once the spinal cord (in this example) has developed, there is no going back[238-244] — the process is irreversible. So it is that an early life temporal lobe lesion, particularly limbic, has an irreversible effect on further temporal lobe development, further epileptic discharges and further development of a behavior disorder which appears often to be schizophrenic.[245-247] Perhaps this organizer of the temporal cortex is reelin,[248,249] although other options, such as excitotoxicity, must be considered. The behavioral change is why temporal lobe epilepsy was once called psychomotor epilepsy. Van Gogh is described as

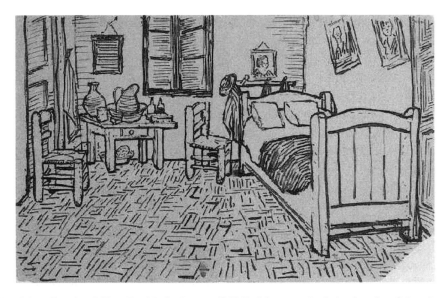

Fig. 16. Sketch of Van Gogh's bedroom (1889). Note particularly the tilt of the picture frames.

having had an early life limbic lesion[245] and a later life behavior disorder, which included amputation of a piece of an ear. Was he hearing bad things? "If thy right eye offend thee" Matthew (5:29:) tells us "pluck it out." His perception, insofar as it is accurately reflected in his painting (Fig. 16), was out of line, tipped, not plumb, as if his vestibular system were involved. These early life temporal lesions have a usual course of a decreasing frequency of seizures and an increasing frequency of interictal behavior disorder, which may be progressive in frequency and in intensity until permanent, as well as an increasing lack of response to the usual anticonvulsant medication. For example, I had a patient, a young woman who had experienced a very early life febrile illness which included seizures. As time went on, her seizures became less frequent and her behavior more disturbed. During the period in her life when she was under my care, she required full-time hospitalization. She was mute except for the occasional word. She wore no clothes; it was impossible to keep her dressed. She displayed no elementary neurological abnormality and had a persistent habit of drinking out of toilet bowls, no matter how much and what was available to drink from more conventional sources. During the years I took care of her, she had a single seizure.

Between these two extremes, there is a third type of temporal lobe epilepsy often alleged to be the typical example. As evident from the two patients described above, typicality is as much a matter of hospital setting in which the patient is seen as it is of the disorder itself. These patients are classically described as being hyper-graphic, hyper-religious and hyposexual. The last of the three is a social construct which is difficult to define. I see the other two as representing a limbic-generated feeling: inchoate, ineffable. The limbic system is a relatively early neurological acquisition in the development of the individual. It precedes the development of isocortex and the development of language. Therefore limbic-generated affect often has no language to express it; the feelings are prelinguistic. The constant writing of the hyper-graphic is in an effort to find the words to express the inexpressible, which perhaps can be expressed only through the ecstasy of religion.

These three kinds of patients all have temporal lobe epilepsy. The difference of expression is a result of different maturational chronology. The early life lesion may produce a behavioral appearance similar to that of schizophrenia, suggesting that the vestibular and other cortex may never have matured properly. The late-life lesion may cause a seizure syndrome with little alteration in interictal behavior because the vestibular representation in cortex reached full maturation before the development of the epileptogenic lesion. To be clear about the speculation, the suggestion is not that the early life lesion causes an aberrant development of the cortex. The suggestion is that the early life temporal lobe seizures may have a deleterious effect on immature nerve cells, perhaps secondary to excitotoxicity. It is known that glutamate is the main excitatory transmitter of the central nervous system and that glutamate (or seizures) in excess can be toxic to nerve cells. The suggestion is that the immature nerve cells — many regions of cortex mature long after birth — are especially vulnerable to intense activity. Their early death precludes normal cortical development. The vulnerability of the immature cell has been ascribed to such things as electrotonic coupling between neurons, inadequate potassium buffering by immature glia, and decreased glucose transport across the blood brain barrier.[250] "…Structural brain damage alone cannot account for the genesis of psychosis."[251]

It has been argued that temporal lobe epilepsy of the dominant temporal lobe is associated with schizophrenic symptoms[80] and the early life acquisition of the cause is emphasized by the report of medial temporal sclerosis in 41 of the 88 patients who underwent temporal lobectomy for intractable epilepsy. Medial temporal sclerosis is thought to occur at the time of delivery. The remaining 47 patients exhibited hamartomas, so-called alien tissue, which is a prenatal abnormality. Thirteen of the 88 had schizophrenia.[251] Twenty-two percent of epileptics with schizophrenic symptoms were left-handed, suggesting an abnormality in the left or dominant hemisphere[110]; note is made of an astonishing 71% of left-handed patients in a group of temporal lobe epileptics with schizophrenia. The inverse relation between overt seizures and psychotic behavior is reaffirmed.[80] That temporal lobe epilepsy produces schizophrenic symptoms does not mean that the cause of schizophrenia is temporal lobe epilepsy or that the cause of schizophrenia resides in the temporal lobe. The cause may relate to a system that includes or terminates in temporal lobe. Interestingly, one such system which has other evidence of involvement — such as eye movement abnormality which does not originate in temporal lobe — is the vestibular, but the evidence for the inclusion of the temporal lobe and of temporal lobe epilepsy in the spectrum of schizophrenic symptomatology is strong.

Does this mean that temporal lobe epilepsy and schizophrenia are related? Only in this sense:

1. The manifestations of temporal lobe epilepsy may be mistaken for the manifestations of schizophrenia.
2. Both may correlate with structural abnormality in the temporal lobe as seen in schizophrenia on imaging studies and may be seen in some cases of temporal lobe epilepsy.
3. The hypothesis is that in both disorders, the final (cortical) projection of the vestibular system is involved whether from a cortical process — temporal lobe epilepsy — or from an abnormality considerably farther downstream in the vestibular system, as in schizophrenia.
4. If the morphological changes in temporal lobe in schizophrenia represent early life loss of temporal lobe neurons and their associated neuropil and if the vestibular system is hyperactive in schizophrenia (whether end organ, nuclei or feedback from the reticular formation), the possibility of early life excitotoxicity for the still immature cortical temporal lobe neurons would parallel the excitotoxicity caused by the early life cortical discharge of epilepsy. Bear in mind that lower levels of the nervous system mature earlier than the cortex, so brain stem reticular formation or vestibular nuclei could generate excitotoxic discharges to the cortex.
5. Auditory hallucinations may occur in both disorders. The epileptic aura may consist of voices or of music. Penfield produced auditory hallucinations by stimulating areas (to judge from his diagrams) quite close to, or actually in, the vestibular area.

Ironically, electroconvulsive therapy has been used in the treatment of schizophrenia with some alleged success, as it has been noted to alleviate some symptoms of Parkinson's disease.

Chapter 9

CONCLUSION

The thesis (really hypothesis) is as follows:

1. The vestibular system is a very old system.
2. It is widely distributed in the brain and the spinal cord.
3. It receives input from the labyrinth, which transmits information about movement and position.
4. Like all sensory systems, it receives feedback which controls its excitability and its gain.
5. Like all sensory systems which relate the organism to the environment, it distributes two types of input. One is specific — that is, it conveys vestibular information to higher levels and enters into reflex behavior, particularly with respect to eye movement. The second is nonspecific and like nonspecific information from other sensory systems, it is projected to the brain stem ascending reticular activating system to serve the function of arousal.
6. Unlike most other sensory systems in which the specific and the nonspecific work in parallel at their first station (that is, when the gain or amplitude of one is raised, the gain of the second is raised), the vestibular system is a tonic system which, at the first stage can dissociate the information provided by its specific input from the information provided by its nonspecific system.
7. The output from the specific system is the output of a null indicator. When the tonic discharge of the labyrinth or vestibular nuclei on one side is balanced by the discharge on the opposite side, movement is not perceived no matter how high or how low the tonic discharge is set. Only when the algebraic sum of the discharge on each side is other than zero, is movement perceived. This constitutes the specific output which is transmitted from the vestibular system to the motor nuclei for eye movement by what can be construed as its lemniscal system — the well-myelinated bundle called the medial longitudinal fasciculus.

8. The nonspecific output is widely distributed in the brain stem to the nuclei of the arousal system. It has been termed the most important contributor other than pain to the arousal mechanism.

9. Projections that are neither connected to the arousal system nor to the ocular reflex system are distributed to the spinal cord, the thalamus, the basal ganglia and the cortex.

10. Distribution in the thalamus is widespread, involving at least ten nuclei excluding the nonspecific intralaminar nuclei. This is very different from the thalamic representation of most other sensory systems. It is probably a reflection of the primacy (early evolutionary development) of vestibular input, which consequently utilized reticular fibers that antedated the appearance of lemnisci.

11. The diffuse thalamic representation probably correlates with the widespread cortical representation of vestibular input. A corollary of this is that unlike other sensory projections, there is nothing that can be legitimately called a primary cortical projection area as there is for vision, hearing, and somatic sensation.

12. This is simply another way of saying that vestibular input is not one of the five classical senses. Still, it is important in perception where its contribution is by the intercession of other senses — particularly vision. To say it differently, the widespread cortical distribution of vestibular input indicates that many of the other cortical sensory areas to which it projects are multimodal, and vestibular input is one of the modes.

13. Insofar as a particularly well-circumscribed region of vestibular cortex has been localized in humans, it is near or overlaps with the auditory region of temporal lobe and the second sensory area of insula.

14. Projections of vestibular nuclei to the spinal cord and the basal ganglia mediate posture and tone. The lateral vestibulospinal tract, terminating on the alpha motor neuron as well as on internuncials, is important for extensor innervation. Extension is represented throughout the vestibular projections and is seen particularly well in the globus pallidus, lesions of which produce flexed postures.

15. The vestibule has intimate connections with the cerebellum as both developed from the same embryonic region. Fibers come directly from the labyrinth as well as from the vestibular nuclei and are distributed in the flocculonodular lobe (the so-called vestibular cerebellum), the anterior and the posterior cerebellar vermis.

16. Parkinson's disease and schizophrenia can be viewed as two sides of the same coin, suggesting that the same neurological systems may be involved in each disorder. In schizophrenia, the input systems seem to

be overactive, while in Parkinson's disease, the input system seems to be deficient.

17. Many things implicate the vestibular system in these two disorders. Most prominent in both are the abnormalities of spontaneous eye movement, the impairment of vestibular testing (not necessarily indicating an end organ locus), the abnormality of posture or tone and the abnormality of sleep patterns (the other side of arousal). Parkinson's disease is also characterized by other signs of affection of the vestibular system including flexed posture, rigid tone and a multitude of eye signs.

18. Perception is claimed to be distorted in schizophrenia. The distortion is not of one of the classic modalities, but is usually of vision in a non-visual sense. The rectitude of the image is distorted as if the vestibular contribution to the visual percept were impaired. The environment is described as "tipped", "wavy" or "uneven". If the observer moves, perceptual symptoms worsen as if stimulating the labyrinth increased perceptual distortion. Patients are said to become immobile, leading to catatonia.

19. Mental changes occur in both disorders and contrast one with the other. The flight of ideas in schizophrenia contrasts with the obsessive thinking of Parkinson's disease. Loose associations of schizophrenia are matched by the rigid compulsive behavior of Parkinson's disease. The hyperattentive state of the schizophrenic is offset by the apathy and lack of initiative of the Parkinsonian. The contrast is between the positive symptoms of schizophrenia and the negative symptoms of Parkinson's disease.

20. If the positive form of schizophrenia reflects hyperactivity of the vestibular input to the ascending reticular activating system, the negative form of the disorder presumably reflects hypoactivity of vestibular input, without the implication of lack of input or lack of transmission. The effect may be the result of an inhibitory process (which is neural activity or excitation) operating at a different level.

21. The similarity between the symptomatology of Parkinson's disease and the negative symptoms of schizophrenia is striking. Apathy, lack of initiative, blunted affect, perseveration of posture and rigidity of muscle tone, most apparent in catatonia, is probably more than coincidence, particularly when one observes that echolalia and echopraxia occur in both disorders.

22. Perhaps the catatonic form of the disorder is the result of focal inhibition without the implication of structural damage known to occur in Parkinson's disease. The question becomes: How does the inhibition get focused? That these negative symptoms are dynamic is evidenced by

the recovery (and the recurrence) of catatonic episodes as well as the occurrence of manic hyperactive catatonia.

23. Is it coincidence that the outstanding imaging abnormality in schizophrenia is atrophy of the cerebellar vermis and that the cerebellar vermis receives from and projects to the vestibular system? Cortical regions in the cerebrum, particularly the temporal vestibular regions, also show imaging abnormalities, but cortical areas project via the pons to the cerebellum. Which came first, the cerebellar or the cortical changes?

24. Purkinje cell function is inhibitory. If vermis atrophy signals Purkinje cell loss, the vestibular nuclei, which receive direct Purkinje cell input, would be disinhibited. The cerebellar fastigial nuclei, which facilitate vestibular nuclear function, would be disinhibited. The combined outcome would be increased excitatory output of the vestibular nuclei to the ascending reticular activating system, increased arousal, hyperattentive behavior and the development of the positive signs and symptoms of schizophrenia.

25. Alternatively, if a large contingent of Purkinje cells is uninvolved in the pathologic process (atrophy) projections from the vestibular system, and from the corticopontocerebellar projections by way of mossy fibers to granule cells, followed by parallel fibers which stimulate large ranks of Purkinje cells, it could initiate a massive inhibitory output, ultimately feeding back to the activating system, causing all the negative symptoms of schizophrenia, including catatonia.

26. Hallucinations, which occur in Parkinson's disease and schizophrenia, differ in that the former tends to be visual, the latter, auditory, although there may be components of each in either disorder. Most hallucinations are visual (including dreaming in the normal), so an obvious question is why schizophrenia hallucinations are usually auditory. If a hyperactive vestibular system plays a role, it is of interest that at the lowest level, there is an anastomosis between the vestibular and auditory systems, raising the possibility that the auditory hallucination may be generated at the first stage of input.

27. An alternative explanation is that the hallucination is actually an illusion induced by an overactive arousal system. Because of heightened arousal, the schizophrenic patient sees and hears things that do not reach conscious awareness in the normal. For most, these environmental stimuli are intrusive and are thus suppressed. For the patient who is hyperalert, these stimuli intrude, reach awareness, and are operated upon by the nervous system to have structure or a meaning imposed on them.

This still leaves the question of why the stimuli should be auditory and strengthens the suspicion for crosstalk between the auditory and the vestibular systems.

28. Whether the hallucination is internally or externally generated, two questions must be explored: (1) Is hallucination a fully formed percept? (2) Does the verbal report of the hallucination accurately reflect the percept? It may not be possible to get an answer to the first question, for all we have to go on is what the patient reports. However, the vagueness of the report ("bad things") makes me wonder whether the experience is of an amorphous or poorly developed sensory (say auditory) input accompanied by a limbic-derived feeling tone. The combination is construed by the patient as "bad things", but the actual words are never provided. If this formulation is correct, the second question is answered. The report does not accurately reflect the percept; it reflects the operation of the nervous system on the unstructured or the poorly structured sensory input to form a coherent, and therefore acceptable, percept.

29. That same sort of operation could explain the genesis of paranoid ideation. The hyperattentive state fragments whole percepts into components. Distinctive features are not recognized and a coherent unity becomes an unrelated collection of fragments. To contain them, control them, put boundaries around them, meaning is imposed from without, just as the way meaning ("bad things") is imposed from without on the sensory fragments that form the hallucination. Hallucination and paranoid ideation may be two aspects of the same phenomenon. The difference is imposed by the normal evaluator because one consists of a "normal" sensory phenomenon (voices, for example) and the other of a "non-normal", "non-sensory" phenomenon (rays, cosmic forces). Suppose they are both composed of an inexpressible limbic feeling, expressed through the medium of unstructured sensory phenomena which become "voices" in hallucination or ideas in paranoia. Those rays and radiowaves must be felt somewhere, otherwise how would the possessor (or the possessed) know they exist? It's a feeling, it's indescribable, it's limbic, (it's like temporal lobe epilepsy) it comes first. In order to control it, we can name it ("radiowaves") and explain it. Hallucinations and paranoia are not fundamentally different; the difference comes from the sensory system used to express them, which is one of the five classical senses for hallucinations — an inexpressible limbic sense for paranoia.

There is still a lot to be done, some of which, perhaps, can explore further the proposal about the vestibular system. In the end, we return, in true sonata form, to where we started, with the words of James Parkinson:

> Should the necessary information be thus obtained, the writer will repine at no censure which the precipitate publication of mere conjectural suggestions may incur; but shall think himself fully rewarded by having excited the attention of those, who may point out the most appropriate means of relieving a tedious and most distressing malady.[1]

APPENDIX

The contention that hallucinations do not exist, but are actually illusions, evokes an understandable skepticism, so engrained is the notion of hallucinations in our culture. In one sense this is nothing but a remnant of Cartesian dualism, for a hallucination is a product of mind, and an illusion, a reaction of body: the opposition of conception and sensation. The problem, of course, is to obtain objective evidence of the stimulus that elicits that response. If the hyperalert nervous system of the patient responds to an environmental event that the normal nervous system ignores or suppresses, how then to get objective verification of its presence? The patient, in the hyperattentive state, cannot report the distinction between the stimulus (reality) and the reaction to it (hallucination). What is needed is a recovered patient who can look back on the hallucinatory episode from the perspective of rationality. This would be a rare find, but it exists.

Virginia Woolf's literary life was punctuated by episodes of hallucinatory psychosis, between which she was able to function effectively as a sensitive novelist. She acknowledged she has been intermittently "mad" and that she had heard voices and had experienced visions. Between episodes, she could retrieve the experiences and call on them for some of her fictional characters. In *Mrs. Dalloway*, Septimus Warren Smith, returned from the war, has episodes of psychosis in which, like Woolf, he hears things and has visions. In real life, roses play an important role: they decorate his wall paper (if I interpret the text correctly — changing light "on the roses, on the wall paper," p. 211[*]), he sees a jar of roses on the mantle (p. 215) and sees his wife pinning an artificial rose to the side of a hat (p. 217) then moving the rose to improve the hat (p. 221). All of that is reality. Then the "hallucination" came.[†] "He lay back in his chair exhausted... Red flowers grew through his flesh... Music began clanging against the rocks up here. It is a motor horn down in

---

[*] Page numbers refer to the Modern Library edition of 1928.
[†] By permission of the Society of Authors, London.

the street he muttered; but up here is cannoned from rock to rock, divided, met in shocks of sound which rose in smooth columns (that music should be visible was a discovery) and became an anthem, an anthem twined round now by a shepherd boy's piping (that's an old man playing a penny whistle by the public-house, he muttered) which, as the boy stood still came bubbling from his pipe, and then, as he climbed higher, made its exquisite plaint while the traffic passed beneath. The boy's elegy is played among the traffic, thought Septimus. Now he withdraws up into the snows, and roses hang about him — the thick red roses which grow on my bedroom wall, he reminded himself. The music stopped. He had his penny, he reasoned it out, and has gone on to the next public-house." (p. 103)

Back and forth, reality and hallucination, from the pen of one who has been there.

REFERENCES

1. Parkinson, J. *An Essay on the Shaking Palsy*, Sherwood, Neely & Jones, London (1817).
2. Magoun, H.W. *The Waking Brain*, C.C. Thomas, Springfield, Illinois (1948).
3. Magoun, H.W. & Rhines, R. An inhibitory mechanism in the bulbar reticular formation, *Journal of Neurophysiology*, Vol. 9, p. 165–171 (1949).
4. Vandewalle, G., Baltoeau, E., Phillips, C. *et al.* Daytime light exposure dynamically enhances brain responses, *Current Biology*, Vol. 16, p. 795–797 (2006).
5. Bhattacharjee, Y. Is internal timing key to mental health? *Science*, Vol. 317, p. 1488–1490 (2007).
6. Jelliffe, S.E. The mental picture in schizophrenia and in epidemic encephalitis, *American Journal of Psychiatry*, Vol. 6, p. 413–465 (1927).
7. Hyman, S.E. Diagnosing disorders, in *The Best of the Brain from Scientific American*, Bloom, F.E. (Ed.), Dana Press, New York, Washington (2007).
8. Szasz, T. *The Myth of Mental Illness: Foundations of a Theory of Personal Contact*, Harper & Rowe, New York (1984).
9. Shorter, E. *A History of Psychiatry*, John Wiley and Son, New York, p. 276 (1997).
10. Wilkinson, G. Political dissent and 'sluggish' schizophrenia in the Soviet Union, *British Medical Journal*, Vol. 293, p. 641–642 (1986).
11. Lyons, D. Soviet style psychiatry is still alive in the People's Republic, *British Journal of Psychiatry*, Vol. 178, p. 380–381 (2001).
12. Paulus, M.P. Decision making dysfunctions in psychiatry – Altered homeostatic processing, *Science*, Vol. 318, p. 602–606 (2007).
13. Marx, J. Evidence linking DISC1 gene to mental illness builds, *Science*, Vol. 318, p. 1062–1063 (2007).
14. Pennisi, E. Breakthrough of the year human genetic variation, *Science*, Vol. 318, p. 1842–1843 (2007).
15. Sontag, S. Illness as metaphor, *The New York Review of Books*, Vol. 24, No. 21 & 22 (1978).

16. Angst, J. Historical aspects of the dichotomy between manic–depressive disorders and schizophrenia, *Schizophrenia Research*, Vol. 57, p. 5–13 (2002).

17. Peraulta, V., Cuesta, M.J., Serrano, J.F. & Mata, I. The Kahlbaum syndrome: A study of its clinical validity, nosological status, and relationship with schizophrenia and mood disorder, *Comprehensive Psychiatry*, Vol. 38, p. 61–67 (1997).

18. Fink, M. Catatonia in DSM-IV, *Biological Psychiatry*, Vol. 36, p. 431–433 (1994).

19. Raitiere, M.N. Subcortical dysrhythmia and catatonia, *Biological Psychiatry*, Vol. 21, p. 1351–1355 (1986).

20. Jablensky, A. The conflict of the nosologists: views on schizophrenia and manic depressive illness in the early part of the twentieth century, *Schizophrenia Research*, Vol. 39, p. 95–100 (1999).

21. Crow, T.J. Schizophrenia, in *Encyclopedia of Genetics*, Brenners, S. & Miller, J.H. (Eds.), Elsevier Science Inc., p. 1774–1776 (2001).

22. Zubin, J., Oppenheimer, G. & Neugebauer, R. Regeneration theory and the stigma of schizophrenia, *Biological Psychiatry*, Vol. 20, p. 1145–1148 (1984).

23. Lieberman, J.A. Is schizophrenia a neurodegenerative disorder? A clinical and neurobiological perspective, *Biological Psychiatry*, Vol. 46, p. 729–739 (1999).

24. Rosenwasser, A.M. & Turek, F.W. Physiology of the mammalian circadian system, Chapter 29, p. 351–362, in *Principles and Practice of Sleep Medicine*, Kryger, M.H., Roth, T. & Dement, W.C. (Eds.), Elsevier, Philadelphia, (2005).

25. Saper, C.B., Lu, J., Chou, T.C. & Gooley, J. The hypothalamic indicator for circadian rhythms, *Trends in Neuro Science*, Vol. 28, p. 152–157 (2005).

26. Stokkan, K.A., Yamazaki, S., Tei, H. *et al.* Entrainment of the circadian clock in the liver by feeding, *Science*, Vol. 29, p. 490–493 (2001).

27. Gooley, J.J., Lu, J., Fischer, D. & Saper, C.B. A broad role for melanopsin in non-visual photoreception, *The Journal of Neuroscience*, Vol. 23, p. 7093–7106 (2003).

28. Moga, M.M. & Moore, R.W. Organization of neural inputs to the suprachiasmatic nucleus in the rat, *Journal of Comparative Neurology*, Vol. 389, p. 508–534 (1998).

29. Reppert, S.M., Weaver, D.R., Rivkees, S.A. & Stopa, G. Putative melatonin receptors in a human biological clock, *Science*, Vol. 242, p. 78–81 (1988).

30. Moore, R.Y. Neural control of the pineal gland, *Behavioral Brain Research*, Vol. 73, p. 125–130 (1996).

31. Moore, R.Y. & Card, J.P. Intergeniculate leaflet: An anatomically and functionally distinct subdivision of the lateral geniculate complex, *Journal of Comparative Neurology*, Vol. 344, p. 403–430 (2004).

32. Morin, L.P. & Blanchard, J.H. Descending projections of the hamster intergeniculate leaflet: Relationship to the sleep/arousal and visuomotor systems, *Journal of Comparative Neurology*, Vol. 487, p. 204–216 (2005).

33. Gooley, J.J. & Saper, C.B. Anatomy of the mammalian circadian system, Chapter 28, p. 335–350, in *Principles and Practice of Sleep Medicine*, Kryger, M.H., Roth, T. & Dement, W.C. (Eds.), Elsevier, Philadelphia (2005).

34. Vandewalle, G., Schmidt, C., Albouy, G. *et al.* Brain responses to violet, blue and green monochromatic light exposures in humans: Prominent role of blue light and the brainstem, *PloS ONE*, Vol. 2, p. e1247 (2007).

35. Vandewalle, G., Gais, S., Schabus, M. *et al.* Wavelength–dependent modulation of brain responses to a working memory task by daytime light exposure, *Cerebral Cortex*, Vol. 17, p. 2788–2795 (2007).

36. Vandewalle, G., Balteau, E., Phillips, C. *et al.* Daytime light exposure dynamically enhances brain responses, *Current Biology*, Vol. 16, p. 1616–1621 (2006).

37. Perrin, F., Peigneux, P., Fuchs, S. *et al.* Nonvisual responses to light exposure in the human brain during the circadian night, *Current Biology*, Vol. 14, p. 1842–1846 (2004).

38. Yoshida, K., McCormack, S., España, R.A. *et al.* Afferents to the orexin neurons of the rat brain, *Journal of Comparative Neurology*, Vol. 494, p. 845–861 (2005).

39. Moruzzi, G. & Magoun, H.W. Brainstem reticular formation and activation of the EEG, *Electroencephalography and Clinical Neurophysiology*, Vol. 1, p. 455–473 (1949).

40. Starzl, T.E., Taylor, C.W. & Magoun, H.W. Collateral afferent excitation of the reticular formation of the brainstem, *Journal of Neurophysiology*, Vol. 14, p. 479–496 (1951).

41. Lu, J., Jhou, T.C. & Saper, C.B. Identification of the wake-active dopaminergic neurons in the ventral periaqueductal brain matter, *Journal of Neuroscience*, Vol. 26, p. 193–202 (2006).

42. Fuller, P.M., Gooley, J.J. & Saper, C.B. Neurobiology of the sleep-wake cycle: sleep architecture, circadian regulation and regulatory feedback, *Journal of Biological Rhythms*, Vol. 21, p. 482–493 (2006).

43. Henny, P. & Jones, B.E. Innervation of the orexin/hypocretin neurons by GABEergic, glutamatergic or cholinergic basal forebrain terminals evidenced by immunostaining for presynaptic vesicular transporter and post synaptic scaffolding protein, *Journal of Comparative Neurology*, Vol. 499, p. 645–661 (2006).

44. Economo, C.V. Sleep as a problem of localization, *Journal of Nervous and Mental Diseases*, Vol. 71, p. 1–5 (1930).

45. Deurvilher, S. & Semba, K. Indirect projections from the suprachiasmatic nucleus to major arousal-promoting cell groups in rat: Implications for the circadian control of behavioral states, *Neuroscience*, Vol. 130, p. 165–183 (2005).

46. Fuller, P.M., Saper, C.B. & Lu, J. The pontine REM switch: Past and present, *Journal of Neurophysiology*, Vol. 584, p. 735–741 (2007).

47. Metts, B.A., Kaufman, G.D. & Perachio, A.A. Polysynaptic inputs to vestibular efferent neurons as revealed by viral transneuronal tracing, *Experimental Brain Research*, Vol. 172, p. 261–274 (2006).

48. Nieuwenhuys, R. The greater limbic system, the emotional motor system, and the brain, Chapter 33, in *Progress in Brain Research*, Vol. 107, p. 551–580 (1996).

49. Jelliffe, S.E. Psychological components in post-encephalitic oculogyric crises, *Archives of Neurology and Psychiatry*, Vol. 21, p. 491–532 (1929).

50. Richter, R. Degeneration of the basal ganglia in monkeys from chronic carbon disulfide poisoning, *Journal of Neuropathology*, Vol. 4, p. 324–353 (1945).

51. Olanow, C.W. Manganese-induced Parkinsonism and Parkinson's disease, *Annals of the New York Academy of Science*, Vol. 1012, p. 209–223 (2004).

52. Stephens, A., Logina, I., Liguts, V. *et al*. A Parkinsonian syndrome in methcathinone users and the role of manganese, *New England Journal of Medicine*, Vol. 358, p. 1009–1017 (2008).

53. Helmsmoortel, J. & vanBogaert, L. Recherches Sur L'Etat des Fonctions Vestibulaires, *Revue Neurologiques*, Vol. 1, p. 980–989 (1927).

54. Dickman, M.S. von Economo Encephalitis, *Archives of Neurology*, Vol. 58, p. 1696–1698 (2001).

55. Gamboa, E.T., Wolf, A., Yahr, M.D. *et al*. Influenza virus antigen in postencephalitic Parkinsonism brain, *Archives of Neurology*, Vol. 31, p. 228–232 (1974).

56. Casals, J., Elizan, T.S. & Yahr, M.D. Postencephalitic Parkinsonism, a review, *Journal of Neural Transmission*, Vol. 105, p. 645–676 (1998).

57. Dale, R.C., Church, A.J., Surtees, R.A.H. *et al*. Encephalitis lethargica syndrome: 20 new cases and evidence of basal ganglia autoimmunity, *Brain*, Vol. 127, p. 21–33 (2004).

58. Wenning, G.K., Jellinger, K. & Litvan, I. Supranuclear gaze palsy and eyelid apraxia in postencephalitic Parkinsonism, *Journal of Neural Transmission*, Vol. 104, p. 845–865 (1997).

59. J.F.F. Food for Thought, *Science*, Vol. 318, p. 1527 (2007) (Abstracted from the *Journal of Biological Chemistry*, Vol. 282, p. 34479 (2007).

60. Schilder, P. The vestibular apparatus in neurosis and psychosis, *Journal of Nervous and Mental Disease*, Vol. 78, p. 1–23, 137–164 (1933).

61. Braak, H., Ghebremedhin, E., Rüb, U. *et al*. Stages in the development of Parkinson's disease-related pathology, *Cell Tissue Research*, Vol. 318, p. 121–134 (2004).

62. Reynolds, L.M. & Locke, S. Relationship between handedness and the side of onset in postencephalitic Parkinsonism, *The Lancet*, Vol. 2, p. 714 (1971).

63. Henneman, E. Relation between size of neurons and their susceptibility to discharge, *Science*, Vol. 126, p. 1345–1347 (1957).

64. Henneman, E., Somjen, G. & Carpenter, D.O. Functional significance of the cell size in spinal motorneurons, *Journal of Neurophysiology*, Vol. 28, p. 560–580 (1965).

65. Henneman, E., Somjen, G. & Carpenter, D.O. Excitability and inhibitability of motorneurons of different sizes, *Journal of Neurophysiology*, Vol. 28, p. 600–620 (1965).

66. Martin, J.P. & Hurwitz, L.J. Locomotion and the basal ganglia, *Brain*, Vol. 85, p. 261–276 (1962).

67. Martin, J.P. & Hurwitz, L.J., Finlayson, M.H. The negative symptoms of basal ganglia disease, *The Lancet*, Vol. 2, p. 62–66 (1962).

68. Schaefer, K.P., & Meyer, D.L. Compensation of vestibular lesions, Chapter 11, p. 463–485, in *Handbook of Sensory Physiology Vestibular System Part 2*, Kornhuber, H.H. (Ed.), Springer-Verlag, New York (1974).

69. Smith, J.L. *Optokinetic Nystagmus*, C.C. Thomas, Springfield, Illinois (1963).

70. Melville-Jones, G. & deJong, J.D. Dynamic characteristics of saccadic eye movements in Parkinson's disease, *Experimental Neurology*, Vol. 31, p. 17–31 (1971).

71. Oepen, G. Association of tardive dyskinesia with increased frequency of eye movements, *European Archives of Psychiatry and Clinical Neuroscience*, Vol. 239, p. 241–245 (1990).

72. Arnulf, I., Konofal, E., Merino-Andreu *et al.* Parkinson's disease and sleepiness, *Neurology*, Vol. 58, p. 1019–1024 (2002).

73. Arnulf, I., Bonnet, A.M., Damier, P. *et al.* Hallucinations, REM sleep and Parkinson's disease, *Neurology*, Vol. 55, p. 281–288 (2000).

74. Mahowald, M.W. & Schenck, C.H. REM sleep parasomnias, Chapter 75, p. 897–916, in *Principles and Practice of Sleep Medicine*, Kryger, M.H., Roth, T & Dement, W.C. (Eds.), Elsevier, Philadelphia (2005).

75. Gagnon, J.F., Bedard, M.A., Fantini, M.L. *et al.* REM sleep behavior disorder and REM sleep without atonia in Parkinson's disease, *Neurology*, Vol. 59, p. 585–589 (2002).

76. Boeve, B.F., Silber, M.H., Parisi, J.E. *et al.* Synucleinopathy pathology and REM sleep behavior disorder plus dementia or Parkinsonism, *Neurology*, Vol. 61, p. 40–45 (2003).

77. Eisensehr, I., Linke, R., Noachtar, S. *et al.* Reduced striatal dopamine transporters in idiopathic rapid eye movement sleep behavior disorder. Comparison with Parkinson's disease and controls, *Brain*, Vol. 24, p. 197–211 (2000).

78. Brodal, A. Anatomy of the vestibular nuclei and their connections, Chapter 1, p. 240–352, in *Handbook of Sensory Physiology, Vestibular System, Part 1*, Kornhuber, H.H. (Ed.), Springer-Verlag, New York (1974).

79. Steriade, M. Brain electrical activity and sensory processing during waking and sleep states, Chapter 9, p. 101–153, in *Principles and Practice of Sleep Medicine*, Kryger, M.H., Roth, T. & Dement W.C. (Eds.), Elsevier, Philadelphia (2005).

80. Flor-Henry, P. Psychosis and temporal lobe epilepsy, a controlled investigation, *Epilepsia*, Vol. 10, p. 363–395 (1969).

81. Bleuler, E. *Dementia Precox or the Group of Schizophrenias* (1911). Translated by Joseph Zinkin, International Universities Press, Madison, Connecticut, p. 9, (1950).

82. Weller, L. & Weller, A. Human menstrual synchrony: A critical assessment, *Neuroscience and Biobehavioral Reviews*, Vol. 17, p. 427–439 (1993).

83. Weller, L., Weller, A., Koresh-Kamin, H. & Ben-Shoshan, R. Menstrual synchrony in a sample of working women, *Psychoneuroendocrinology*, Vol. 24, p. 449–459 (1999).

84. Williams, R.L., Karacan, I. & Hursch, C.J. *Electroencephalography of Human Sleep: Clinical Applications*, John Wiley, New York (1974).

85. Patterson, P.H. Maternal effects on schizophrenia risk, *Science*, Vol. 318, p. 576–577 (2007).

86. Haroutunian, V. & Davis, K.L. Myelin and oligodendrocyte abnormalities in schizophrenia, *International Journal of Neuropsychopharmacology*, Vol. 10, p. 499–502 (2007).

87. Wade, N. First gene for social behavior identified in whiskery mice, *The New York Times* (September 9, 1997).

88. Kozlovsky, N., Belmaker, R.H. & Agam, G. GSK-3 and the neurodevelopmental hypothesis of schizophrenia, *European Neuropsychopharmacology*, Vol. 12, p. 13–25 (2002).

89. Impagnatiello, F., Guidotti, A.R., Pesold, C. *et al.* A decrease of reelin expression as a putative vulnerability function in schizophrenia, *Proceedings of the National Academy of Science*, Vol. 95, p. 15718–15723 (1998).

90. Guidotti, A.R., Auta, J., Davis, J.M. *et al.* Decrease in reelin and glutamic acid decarboxylase 67 expression in schizophrenia and bipolar disorder, *Archives of General Psychiatry*, Vol. 57, p. 1061–1069 (2000).

91. Abi-Dargham, A. Do we still believe in the dopamine hypothesis? New data bring new evidence. *International Journal of Neuropsychopharmacology*, Supplement 1, p. S1–S5 (2004).

92. Andreasen, N.C. Schizophrenia: The fundamental questions, *Brain Research Reviews*, 31, p. 106–112 (2000).

93. Miller, D.D., Arndt, S. & Andreasen N.C. Alogia, attentional impairment and inappropriate affect: Their status in the dimensions of schizophrenia, *Comprehensive Psychiatry*, Vol. 34, p. 221–226 (1993).

94. Andreasen, N.C. Symptoms, signs and diagnosis of schizophrenia, *The Lancet*, Vol. 346, p. 477–481 (1995).

95. Kahlbaum, K. Catatonia, Johns Hopkins University Press, Baltimore Maryland (1973).

96. Mettler, F.A. Perceptual capacity, functions of the corpus striatum and schizophrenia, *Psychiatric Quarterly*, Vol. 25, p. 89–111 (1955).

97. Jellife, S.E. The mental pictures in schizophrenia and in epidemic encephalitis, *American Journal of Psychiatry*, Vol. 6, p. 413–465 (1927).

98. Salokangas, R.K.R., Hunkonen, T., Stengard, E. *et al.* Negative symptoms and neuroleptics in catatonic schizophrenia, *Schizophrenia Research*, Vol. 59, p. 73–76 (2003).

99. Magrinat, G., Danzinger, J.A., Lorenzo, I.C. & Flemenbaum, A. A reassessment of catatonia, *Comprehensive Psychiatry*, Vol. 24, p. 218–228 (1983).

100. Baldessarini, R.J. & Lapinski, J.F. Schizophrenia, in *Principles of Internal Medicine* (Harrison's Textbook), 8th Edn., McGraw Hill, New York (1977).

101. Lee, J.W.Y. Chronic catatonia, negative symptoms and response to selegiline and amantadine, *Australian and New Zealand Journal of Psychiatry*, Vol. 39, p. A62 (2005).

102. Javitt, D.C. & Coyle, J.T. Decoding schizophrenia, in *The Best of the Brain from Scientific American*, Bloom, F.E. (Ed.), Dana Press, New York (2007).

103. Mettler, F.A. *Psychosurgical Problems*, by the Columbia Graystone Associates, The Blakiston Company, New York (1952).

104. Mettler, F.A., Crandell, A., Wittenborn, J.R. *et al.* Factors in the preoperative situation of schizophrenics considered to be of significance in influencing the outcome following psychosurgery, *Psychiatric Quarterly*, Vol. 28, p. 549–606 (1954).

105. Chapman, J. The early symptoms of schizophrenia, *British Journal of Psychiatry*, Vol. 112, p. 225–251 (1966).

106. Previc, F.H. A 'neuropsychology of schizophrenia' without vision, *Behavioral and Brain Sciences*, Vol. 16, p. 207–208 (1993).

107. Maher, B.A. A tentative theory of schizophrenic utterance, *Progress in Experimental Personality Research*, Vol. 12, Academic Press, New York (1983).

108. Shimkunas, A. Hemispheric asymmetry and schizophrenic thought disorder, in *Language and Cognition in Schizophrenia*, Schwartz, S. (Ed.), Lawrence Erlbaum Associates, New York (1978).

109. Locke, S., Caplan, D. & Kellar, L. *A Study in Neurolinguistics*, C.C. Thomas, Springfield, Illinois (1973).

110. Flor-Henry, P. Psychopathology and hemispheric specialization: Left hemisphere dysfunction in schizophrenia, psychopathy, hysteria and the obsessional syndrome, Chapter 22, p. 477–494, in *Handbook of Neuropsychology*, Vol. 3, Squire, L. & Gianotti, G. (Eds.), Elsevier, New York (1989).

111. Witkin, H.A., Lewis, H.B., Hertzman, M. *et al. Personality through Perception*, Harper and Brothers, New York (1954).

112. Ornitz, E.M. Vestibular dysfunction in schizophrenia and childhood autism, *Comprehensive Psychiatry*, Vol. 11, p. 159–173 (1970).

113. Diefendorf, A.R. & Dodge, R. An experimental study of the ocular reactions of the insane for photographic records, *Brain*, Vol. 31, p. 453–489 (1908).

114. Warren, S. & Ross, R.G. Deficient cancellation of the vestibular ocular reflex in schizophrenia, *Schizophrenia Research*, Vol. 34, p. 187–193 (1998).

115. Holzman, P.S. Eye movements and the search for the essence of schizophrenia, *Brain Research Reviews*, Vol. 31, p. 350–356 (2000).

116. Odaira, N., Yamada, T., Tsukamoto, Y., Kawano, H., Anezaki, R. & Tani, M. Vestibular function in schizophrenia, *Bulletin of Allied Medical Sciences*, Kobe, Vol. 7, p. 77–82 (1991).

117. Park, S., Lenzenweger, M.F., Puschel, J. & Holzman, P. Attentional inhibition in schizophrenia and schizotypy, A spatial negative priming study, *Cognitive Neuropsychology*, Vol. 1, p. 125–149 (1996).

118. McGhie, A. & Chapman, J. Disorders of attention and perception in early schizophrenia, *British Journal of Medical Physiology*, Vol. 34, p. 103–116 (1961).

119. Shakow, D. Segmental set: A theory of the formal psychological deficit in schizophrenic, *Archives of General Psychiatry*, Vol. 6, p. 1–17 (1962).

120. Elkins, I.J. & Cromwell, R.L. Priming effects in schizophrenia, *Journal of Abnormal Psychology*, Vol. 103, p. 791–800 (1994).

121. Nestor, P.G., Fauz, S.F., McCarley, R.W., Penhune, V., Shenton, M.E. *et al.* Attentional cues in chronic schizophrenia, *Journal of Abnormal Psychology*, Vol. 101, p. 682–689 (1992).

122. Holzman, P.D., Levy, D. & Proctor, L. The several qualities of attention in schizophrenia, in *The Nature of Schizophrenia*, Wynne, L. (Ed.), John Wiley, New York (1978).

123. Collins, W.E. Manipulation of arousal and its effects on human vestibular nystagmus induced by caloric irrigation and angular accelerations, *Aerospace Medicine*, p. 124–129 (February 1963).

124. Fitzgerald, G. & Stengel, E. Vestibular reactivity to caloric stimulation in schizophrenics, *Journal of Mental Sciences*, Vol. 91, p. 93–100 (1945).

125. Baruk, C.H. & Aubry, M. Contribution au L'Etude de la Demence Precoce Catatonique; Excitabilite Labrynthique au Cours de la Catatonie, *Rev. Neurol.*, Vol. 1, p. 976–980 (1927).

126. Angyal, A. & Blackman, N. Vestibular reactivity in schizophrenia, *Archives of Neurology and Psychiatry*, Vol. 44, p. 611–620 (1940).

127. Jones, A.M. & Pivik, R.T. Vestibular activation, smooth pursuit tracking, and psychosis, *Psychiatry Research*, Vol. 14, p. 291–308 (1985).

128. Blackwood, D.H.R., Ebmeier, K.P., Muir, W.J. *et al.* Correlation of regional cerebral blood flow equivalents measured by single photon emission computerized tomography with P300 latency and eye movement abnormality in schizophrenia, *Acta psychiatrica scandinavica*, Vol. 990, p. 157–166 (1994).

129. Clementz, B.A., McDowell, J.E. & Zisook, S. Saccadic system functioning among schizophrenic patients and their first-degree biological relatives, *Journal of Abnormal Psychology*, Vol. 103, p. 277–287 (1994).

130. Shuster, A.R. The psychotropic drugs: Considerations relative to the vestibular pathways and testing, *The Laryngoscope*, Vol. 75, p. 707–749 (1965).

131. Robinson, D.A. Vestibular and optokinetic symbiosis, in *Control of Gaze by Brainstem Neurons*, Baker, R. & Bertoz, A. (Eds.), Elsevier, New York (1977).

132. Latham, C., Holzman, P.S., Manschreck, T.C. & Tole, J. Optokinetic nystagmus and pursuit eye movements in schizophrenia, *Archives of General Psychiatry*, Vol. 38, p. 997–1003 (1981).

133. Schifferli, P. L'Examen du Nystagmus Optocinétique Dans la Schizophrénie, *Schweizerische Medizinische Wochenschrift*, Vol. 87, p. 1143–1145 (1957).

134. Lipper, S. Impairment of optokinetic nystagmus in patients with tardive dyskinesia, *Archives of General Psychiatry*, Vol. 28, p. 331–333 (1973).

135. Wertheim, A.H., vanGelder, P., Lautin, A. *et al.* High thresholds for movement perception in schizophrenia may indicate abnormal extraneous noise levels of central vestibular activity, *Biological Psychiatry*, Vol. 20, p. 1197–1210 (1985).

136. Wertheim, A.H. Motion perception during self motion: The direct versus inferential controversy revisited, *Behavioral and Brain Sciences*, Vol. 17, p. 293–311 (1994).

137. Schmahmann, J.D. *The Cerebellum and Cognition*, Academic Press, New York (1997).

138. Yeterian, E.H. & Pandya, D.N. Striatal connections of the parietal association cortices in rhesus monkeys, *The Journal of Comparative Neurology*, Vol. 332, p. 175–197 (1993).

139. Nishino, S., Ripley, B., Mignot, E. *et al.* CSF hypocretin-1 levels in schizophrenics and controls: Relationship to sleep architecture, *Psychiatry Research*, Vol. 110, p. 1–7 (2002).

140. Keshavan, M.S., Reynolds, C.F., Miewald, J.M. *et al.* Delta sleep deficits in schizophrenia, *Archives of General Psychiatry*, Vol. 55, p. 443–448 (1998).

141. Ferrarelli, F., Huber, R., Peterson, M.J. *et al.* Reduced sleep spindle activity in schizophrenia patients, *American Journal of Psychiatry*, Vol. 164, p. 483–492 (2007).

142. Ganguli, R., Reynolds, C.F. & Kupfer, D.J. Electroencephalographic sleep in the young, never medicated schizophrenics, *Archives of General Psychiatry*, Vol. 44, p. 36–44 (1987).

143. Kato, M., Kajimura, N., Okuma, T. *et al.* Association between delta waves during sleep and negative symptoms in schizophrenia, *Neuropsychobiology*, Vol. 39, p. 165–172 (1999).
144. Lauer, C.J., Schreiber, W., Pollmacher, T. *et al.* Sleep in schizophrenia: A polysomnographic study on drug naive patients, *Neuropsychopharmacology*, Vol. 16, p. 51–60 (1997).
145. Carskadon, M.A. & Rechtschaffen, A. Monitoring and staging human sleep, Chapter 116, p. 1359–1377, in *Principles and Practice of Sleep Medicine*, Kryger, M.H., Roth, T. & Dement, W.C. (Eds.), Elsevier, Philadelphia (2005).
146. Steriade, M. Brain electrical activity and sensory processing during waking and sleep states, Chapter 9, p. 101–119, in *Principles and Practice of Sleep Medicine*, Kryger, M.H., Roth, T. & Dement, W.C. (Eds.), Elsevier, Philadelphia (2005).
147. Zarcone, V., Gulevich, G., Pivik, T. & Dement, W. Partial REM phase deprivation and schizophrenia, *Archives of General Psychiatry*, Vol. 18, p. 194–202 (1968).
148. Pompeiano, O. & Somogyi, I. Spontaneous activity of single vestibular neurons of unrestrained cats during sleep and wakefulness, *Archives Italiennes de Biologie*, Vol. 102, p. 308–330 (1964).
149. Pompeiano, O. & Morrison, A.R. Vestibular influences during sleep: I. abolition of the rapid eye movements during desynchronized sleep following vestibular lesions, *Archives Italiennes de Biologie*, Vol. 103, p. 569–595 (1965).
150. Hartmann, E. & Cravens, J. Sleep: Effects of *d* and *l* amphetamine in man and in rat *Psychopharmacology*, Vol. 50, p. 171–175 (2004).
151. Nestler, E.J. & Malenka, R.C. The addicted brain, Chapter 13, p. 142–155, *The Best of the Brain from Scientific American*, Bloom, F.E. (Ed.), Dana Press, New York (2007).
152. Nashino, N.S. & Mignot, E. Wake promoting medications, Chapter 38, p. 468–485, in *Principles and Practice of Sleep Medicine*, Kryger, M.H., Roth, T. & Dement, W.C. (Eds.), Elsevier, Philadelphia (2005).
153. Mitler, M.M. & O'Malley, M.B. Wake promoting medications: Efficacy and adverse effects, Chapter 39, p. 484–498, in *Principles and Practice of Sleep Medicine*, Kryger, M.H., Roth, T. & Dement, W.C. (Eds.), Elsevier, Philadelphia (2005).
154. Jones, B.E. Basic mechanics of sleep-wake states, Chapter 11, p. 136–153, in *Principles and Practice of Sleep Medicine*, Kryger, M.H., Roth, T. & Dement, W.C. (Eds.), Elsevier, Philadelphia (2005).
155. Feinberg, I. Schizophrenia: Caused by a fault in programmed synaptic elimination during adolescence? *Journal of Psychiatric Research*, Vol. 17, p. 319–334 (1983).
156. McCarley, R.W., Shenton, M.E., O'Donnell, B.F. *et al.* Auditory P300 abnormalities and left posterior superior temporal gyrus volume reduction in schizophrenia, *Archives of General Psychiatry*, Vol. 50, p. 190–197 (1993).

157. Suddath, R.L., Christison, G.W., Torrey, E.F. *et al.* Anatomical abnormalities in the brains of monozygotic twins discordant for schizophrenia, *New England Journal of Medicine*, Vol. 322, p. 789–794 (1990).

158. Wyser, A.K., Andreasen, N.C., O'Leary, D.S. *et al.* Dysfunctional corticocerebellar circuits cause 'cognitive dysmetria' in schizophrenia, *Neurology Report*, Vol. 9, p. 1895–1899 (1998).

159. Sears, L.L., Andreasen, N.C. & O'Leary, D.S. Cerebellar functional abnormalities in schizophrenia are suggested by classical eyeblink conditioning, *Biological Psychiatry*, Vol. 48, p. 204–209 (2000).

160. Postrel, V. Playing to type, *The Atlantic*, p. 143–146 (2008).

161. Oswald, I. Dreaming, *The Oxford Companion to the Mind*, Gregory, R.L. (Ed.), Oxford University Press, Oxford (1987).

162. Benson, K.L. & Zarcone, V.P. Schizophrenia, Chapter 113, p. 1327–1336, in *Principles and Practice of Sleep Medicine*, Kryger, M.H., Roth, T. & Dement, W.C. (Eds.), Elsevier, Philadelphia (2005).

163. Ribstein, M. Hypnagogic hallucinations, Chapter 8, in *Narcolepsy*, Guilleminault, C., Dement, W.C. & Passouant, P. (Eds.), Spectrum Publications, New York (1975).

164. Ridha, B.H., Josephs, K.A. & Rossor, M.N. Delusions and hallucinations in dementia with Lewy bodies: Worsening with memantine, *Neurology*, Vol. 65, p. 481–482 (2005).

165. Kulisevsky, J. & Roldan, E. Hallucinations and sleep disturbances in Parkinson's disease, *Neurology*, Vol. 63, p. S28–S30 (2004).

166. McKeith, I.G., Dickson, D.W., Lowe, J. *et al.* Diagnosis and management of dementia with Lewy bodies: Third report of the DLB Consortium, *Neurology*, Vol. 65, p. 1863–1872 (2005).

167. Simard, M., van Reekum, R. & Cohen, T. A review of the cognitive and behavioral symptoms in dementia with Lewy bodies, *Journal of Neuropsychiatry Clinical Neuroscience*, Vol. 12, p. 425–450 (2000).

168. Ferman, T.J. Dementia with Lewy bodies: A review of clinical diagnosis, neuropathology and management options, Website: Mayo Clinic, Jacksonville (2000).

169. Zaccai, J., Brayne, C., McKeith, I. *et al.* Patterns and the stages of alpha synucleopathy, *Neurology*, Vol. 70, p. 1042–1048 (2008).

170. Onofrj, M., Thomas, A., D'Andreamatteo, G. *et al.* Incidence of RBD and hallucination in patients affected by Parkinson's disease: Eight year follow-up, *Neurology Science*, Vol. 23, p. S91–S94, (2002).

171. Rechtshaffen, A. & Seigel, J. Sleep and dreaming, Chapter 47, p. 936–947, in *Principles of Neural Science,* 4th Ed., Kandel, E.R., Schwartz, J.H. & Jessel, T.M. (Eds.), McGraw-Hill, New York (1991).

172. Solms, M. Dreaming and REM sleep are controlled by different brain mechanisms, *Behavioral and Brain Sciences*, Vol. 23, p. 793–821 (2000).

173. Solms, M. Freud returns, Chapter 3, in *The Best of the Brain from Scientific American*, Bloom, F.E. (Ed.), Dana Press, New York (2007).

174. Hobson, J.A. Freud returns? Like a bad dream, Chapter 3, in *The Best of the Brain from Scientific American*, Bloom, F.E. (Ed.), Dana Press, New York (2007).

175. Lim, A.S., Lozano, A.M., Moreau, E. *et al.* Characterization of REM-sleep associated ponto-geniculo-occipital waves in the human pons, *Sleep*, Vol. 30, p. 823–827 (2007).

176. Pompeiano, O. & Morrison, A.R. Vestibular input to the lateral geniculate nucleus during desynchronized sleep, *Pflugers Arch Gesamte Physiol Menschen Tiere*, Vol. 290, p. 272–274 (1966).

177. Pompeiano, O. Mechanisms responsible for spinal inhibition during desynchronized sleep: Experimental study, Chapter 25, in *Narcolepsy*, Guilleminault, C., Dement, W.C. & Passouant, P. (Eds.), Spectrum Publications, New York (1975).

178. Hobson, J.A. & Stickgold, R. Dreaming: A neurocognitive approach, *Consciousness and Cognition*, Vol. 3, p. 1–15 (1994).

179. Maquet, P., Peters, J.M., Aerts, J. *et al.* Functional neuroanatomy of human rapid-eye-movement sleep and dreaming, *Nature*, Vol. 383, p. 163–166 (1996).

180. Lovblad, K.O., Thomas, R., Jacob, P.M. *et al.* Silent functional magnetic resonance imaging demonstrates focal activation in rapid eye movement sleep, *Neurology*, Vol. 53, p. 2193–2195 (1999).

181. Maquet, P., Ruby, P., Maudoux, A. *et al.* Human cognition during REM sleep and the activity profile within frontal and parietal cortices: A reappraisal of functional neuroimaging data, *Progress in Brain Research*, Vol. 150, p. 219–227 (2005).

182. Braun, A.R., Balkin, T.J., Wesensten, N.J. *et al.* Dissociated pattern of activity in visual cortices and their projections during human rapid eye movement sleep, *Science*, Vol. 279, p. 91–95 (1998).

183. Nofzinger, E.A. Neuroimaging and sleep medicine, *Sleep Medicine Reviews*, Vol. 9, p. 157–172 (2005).

184. Nofzinger, E.A. Functional neuroimaging of Sleep, *Seminars in Neurology*, Vol. 25, p. 9–16 (2005).

185. Aserinsky, E. & Kleitman, N. Regularly occurring periods of eye motility and concomitant phenomena during sleep, *Science*, Vol. 118, p. 273–274 (1953).

186. Llinas, R. & Ribary, U. Coherent 40-Hz oscillation characterizes dream state in humans, *Proceedings of the National Academy of Science*, Vol. 90, p. 2078–2081 (1993).

187. Brodal, A., Pompeiano, O. & Walberg, F. *The Vestibular Nuclei and their Connections: Anatomy and Functional Correlation*, Oliver and Boyd, London (1962).

188. Kandel, E.R. Disorders of thought and volition, Chapter 60, p. 1188–1208, in *Principles of Neural Science*, 4th Ed., Kandel, E.R., Schwartz, J.H. & Jessel, T.M. (Eds.), McGraw-Hill, New York (1991).

189. Silbersweig, D.A., Stern, E., Frith, C. *et al.* A functional neuroanatomy of hallucinations in schizophrenia, *Nature*, Vol. 378, p. 176–179 (1995).

190. Flor-Henry, P. Psychosis, neurosis and epilepsy, *British Journal of Psychiatry*, Vol. 124, p. 144–150 (1974).

191. Cleghorn, J.M., Franco, S., Szechtman, B. *et al.* Toward a brain map of auditory hallucinations, *American Journal of Psychiatry*, Vol. 149, p. 1062–1069 (1992).

192. Stephane, M., Hagen, M.C., Lee, J.T. *et al.* About the mechanisms of auditory verbal hallucinations: A positron emission tomographic study, *Journal of Psychiatry Neurological Science*, Vol. 31, p. 396–405 (2006).

193. McGuire, P.K., Silbersweig, D.A., Wright, I. *et al.* The neural correlates of inner speech and auditory verbal imagery in schizophrenia: Relationship to auditory verbal hallucinations, *British Journal of Psychiatry*, Vol. 169, p. 148–159 (1996).

194. Akbarian, S., Grusser, O.J. & Guldin, W.O. Thalamic connections of the vestibular cortical fields in the squirrel monkey (Saimiri Sciureus), *Journal of Comparative Neurology*, Vol. 326, p. 423–441 (1992).

195. Frederickson, J.M., Kornhuber, H.H. & Schwarz, D.W.F. Cortical projections of the vestibular nerve, Chapter 6, p. 465–482, in *The Handbook of Sensory Physiology, Vestibular Systems, Part 1*, Kornhuber, H.H. (Ed.), Springer-Verlag, New York (1974).

196. Precht, W. The physiology of the vestibular nuclei, Chapter 2, p. 353–416, in *The Handbook of Sensory Physiology, Vestibular Systems, Part 1*, Kornhuber, H.H. (Ed.), Springer-Verlag, New York (1974).

197. Pompeiano, O. Cerebello-vestibular interrelations, Chapter 3, p. 417–476, in *The Handbook of Sensory Physiology, Vestibular Systems, Part 1*, Kornhuber, H.H. (Ed.), Springer-Verlag, New York (1974).

198. Hallpike, C.S. Some types of ocular nystagmus and their neurological mechanisms, *Proceedings of the Royal Society of Medicine*, Vol. 60, p. 1043–1054 (1967).

199. Wright, S., Hilsz, J. & Locke, S. Medial occipital projections to the nucleus of darkschewitsch of rhesus monkey, *Anatomical Record*, Vol. 178, p. 667–670 (1974).

200. DeKleyn, A. The connections between the optokinetic nystagmus and the vestibular system, *ACTA Otolaryngologica*, S. 78, p. 8–13 (1949).

201. Dix, M.R., Hallpike, C.S. & Harrison, M.S. Experimental observations upon the subcortical pathways of optokinetic and vestibular nystagmus, *Proceedings of the Physiological Society*, p. 22–23 (1949).

202. Precht, W. Physiological aspects of the efferent vestibular system, Chapter 5, p. 221–236, in *The Handbook of Sensory Physiology, Vestibular Systems, Part 1*, Kornhuber, H.H. (Ed.), Springer-Verlag, New York (1974).

203. Horowitz, S.S., Blanchard, J. & Morin, L.P. Medial vestibular connections with the hypocretin (orexin) system, *Journal of Comparative Neurology*, Vol. 487, p. 127–146 (2005).

204. Locke, S. Subcortical projection of the magnocellular medial geniculate nucleus of monkey, *Journal of Comparative Neurology*, Vol. 138, p. 321–328 (1970).

205. Locke, S. The projection of the magnocellular medial geniculate body, *Journal of Comparative Neurology*, Vol. 116, p. 179–193 (1961).

206. Roucoux-Hanus, M. & Boisacq-Schepens, N. Ascending vestibular projections: Further results at cortical and thalamic levels in the cat, *Experimental Brain Research*, Vol. 29, p. 283–292 (1977).

207. Caston, J. & Bricout-Berthout, A. Responses of afferent and efferent neurons to visual inputs in the vestibular nerve of the frog, *Brain Research*, Vol. 240, p. 141–145 (1982).

208. Herrick, C.J. *The Brain of the Tiger Salamander*, University of Chicago Press, Chicago (1948).

209. Weinberger, D.R., Torrey, E.F. & Wyatt, R.J. Cerebellar atrophy in chronic schizophrenia, *The Lancet*, Vol. 1, p. 718–719 (1979).

210. Weinberger, D.R., Kleinman, J.E. & Luchins, D.J. *et al.* Cerebellar pathology in schizophrenia, a controlled postmortem study, *American Journal of Psychiatry*, Vol. 137, p. 359–361 (1980).

211. Schmahmann, J.D. The role of the cerebellum in affect and psychosis, *Journal of Neurolinguistics*, Vol. 13, p. 189–214 (2000).

212. Wassink, T.H., Andreasen, N.C., Nopoulos, P. & Flaum, M. Cerebellar morphology as a predictor of symptom and psychosocial outcome in schizophrenia, *Biological Psychiatry*, Vol. 45, p. 41–48 (1999).

213. Elisevich, K. & Redekop, G. The fastigial pressor response, *Journal of Neurosurgery*, Vol. 74, p. 147–151 (1991).

214. Martin, P., Albers, M. The cerebellum and schizophrenia, a selective review, *Schizophrenia Bulletin*, Vol. 21, p. 241–250 (1995).

215. Saab, C.Y., Garcia-Nicas, E. & Willis, W.D. Stimulation in the rat fastigial nucleus enhances the responses of neurons in the dorsal column nuclei to innocuous stimuli, *Neuroscience Letters*, Vol. 327, p. 17–20 (2002).

216. Ramnani, N. The primate cortico-cerebellar system: Anatomy and function, *Nature Reviews*, Vol. 7, p. 511–522 (2006).

217. Schahmann, J.D., Rosene, D.L. & Pandya, D.N. Motor projections to the basis pontis in rhesus monkey, *Journal of Comparative Neurology*, Vol. 478, p. 248–268 (2004).

218. Daskalakis, Z.J., Christensen, B.K., Fitzgerald, P.B. *et al.* Reduced cerebellar inhibition in schizophrenia, a preliminary study, *American Journal of Psychiatry*, Vol. 162, p. 1203–1205 (2005).

219. Ghez, C. & Thach, W.T. The cerebellum, Chapter 42, p. 832–852 in *Principles of Neural Science*, 4th Ed., Kandel, E.R., Schwartz, J.H. & Jessel, T.M. (Eds.), McGraw-Hill, New York, (1991).

220. Billig, I. & Balaban, C.D. "Zonal Organization of the Vestibulo-Cerebellar Pathways Controls the Horizontal Eye Muscles Using Two Recombinant Strains of Pseudorabies Virus", *Neuroscience*, Vol. 133, p. 1047–1393 (2002).

221. Billig, I. & Balaban, C.D. "Zonal Organization of the Vestibulo-Cerebellar Pathways in the Control of Horizontal Extraocular Muscles Using Pseudorabies Virus: I Flocculus/Ventral Laraflocculus", *Neuroscience*, Vol. 125, p. 507–520 (2004).

222. Kaufman, G.D., Mustari, M.J., Miselis, R.R. & Perachio, A.A. Transneuronal pathways to the vestibulocerebellum, *Journal of Comparative Neurology*, Vol. 370, p. 501–523 (1996).

223. Andre, P., d'Ascanio, P. & Pompeiano, O. Noradrenergic agents into cerebellar anterior vermis modify the gain of vestibulospinal reflexes in the cat, *Progress in Brain Research*, Vol. 88, p. 463–484 (1991).

224. Slater, P., Doyle, C.A. & Deakin, J.F.W. Abnormal persistence of cerebellar serotonin 1A receptors in schizophrenia suggest failure to regress in neonates, *Journal of Neural Transmission*, Vol. 105, p. 305–315 (1998).

225. Wepsic, J.G. Multimodal sensory activation of cells in the magnocellular medial geniculate nucleus, *Experimental Neurology*, Vol. 15, p. 299–318 (1966).

226. Wepsic, J.G. & Sutin, J. Posterior thalamic and septal influence upon pallidal and amygdaloid slow wave and unitary activity, *Experimental Neurology*, Vol. 10, p. 67–80 (1964).

227. Mettler, F.A. & Mettler, C.C. Labyrinthine disregard after removal of the caudate, *Proceedings of the Society Experimental Biology and Medicine*, Vol. 45, p. 473–475 (1940).

228. Muskens, L.J.J. The central connections of the vestibular nuclei with the corpus striatum, and their significance for ocular movements and for locomotion, *Brain*, Vol. 45, p. 454–478 (1922).

229. Shiroyama, T., Kayahara, T., Yasui, Y. *et al.* Projections of the vestibular nuclei to the thalamus in the rat: *A Phaseolus Vulgaris* leukoagglutinin study, *Journal of Comparative Neurology*, Vol. 407, p. 318–332 (1999).

230. DeLong, M.R. The basal ganglia, Chapter 43, p. 853–867 in *Principles of Neural Science,* 4th Ed, Kandel, E.R., Schwartz, J.H. & Jessel, T.M. (Eds.), McGraw-Hill, New York (1991).

231. Horowitz, S.S., Blanchard, J.H. & Morin, L.P. Intergeniculate leaflet and ventral lateral geniculate nucleus afferent connections: An anatomical substrate for functional input from the vestibulo-visuomotor system, *Journal of Comparative Neurology*, Vol. 474, p. 227–245 (2004).

232. Fasold, O., vonBrevern, M., Kuhberg, M. *et al.* Human vestibular cortex as identified with caloric stimulation in functional magnetic resonance imaging, *Neuroimage*, Vol. 17, p. 1384–1393 (2002).

233. Kahane, P., Hoffmann, D., Minotti, L. & Berthoz, A. Reappraisal of the human vestibular cortex by cortical electrical stimulation study, *Annals of Neurology*, Vol. 54, p. 615–624 (2003).

234. Smiley, J.F., Hackett, T.A., Ulbert, I. *et al.* Multisensory convergence in auditory cortex, I. cortical connections of the caudal superior temporal plane in Macaque monkeys, *Journal of Comparative Neurology*, Vol. 502, p. 894–923 (2007).

235. Pandya, D.N., Rosene, D.L. & Doolittle, A.M. Corticothalamic connections of auditory related areas of the temporal lobe in the rhesus monkey, *Journal of Comparative Neurology*, Vol. 345, p. 447–471 (2004).

236. Akbarian, S., Grusser, O.J. & Guldin, W.O. Corticofugal projections to the vestibular nuclei in squirrel monkeys. Further evidence of multiple cortical vestibular fields, *Journal of Comparative Neurology*, Vol. 332, p. 89–104 (1993).

237. Penfield, W. & Jasper, H. *Epilepsy and the Functional Anatomy of the Human Brain*, Little Brown & Company, Boston (1954).

238. Khokha, M., Yeh, J., Grammer, T.C. & Harland, R.M. Depletion of three BMP antagonists from Spemanns' organizer leads to a catastrophic loss of dorsal structures, *Developmental cell*, Vol. 8, p. 401–411 (2005).

239. De Robertis, E.M., Wessely, O., Oelgeschlager, M. *et al.* Molecular mechanisms of cell-cell signaling by the Spemann-Mangold organizer, *International Journal of Developmental Biology*, Vol. 45, p. 189–197 (2001).

240. Hurtado, C. & De Robertis, E.M. Neural induction in the absence of organizer in salamanders is mediated by Ras/Mapk, *Developmental Biology*, Vol. 307, p. 282–289 (2007).

241. Sander, K. & Faessler, P.E. Introducing the Spemann-Mangold organizer: Experiments and insights that generated a key concept in developmental biology, *International Journal of Developmental Biology*, Vol. 45, p. 1–11 (2001).

242. Kumar, A., Godwin, J.W., Gates, P.B. *et al.* Molecular basis for the nerve dependence of limb regeneration in an adult vertebrate, *Science*, Vol. 318, p. 772 (2007).

243. Sanders, R. University of California Berkeley Press Release (March 9, 2005).

244. De Robertis, E.M. Speemann's organizer and self regulation in amphibian embryos, *Nature Reviews Molecular Cell Biology*, published online (1 February 2006).

245. Gastaut, H. La Maladie de Vincent van Gogh Envisagée a la Lumiere des Conceptions Nouvelles Sur L'Epilepsie Psychomotrice, *Annales of Medico-Psychologiques*, Vol. 114, p. 196–237 (1956).

246. Bredkjaer, S.R., Mortensen, P.B. & Parnas, J. Epilepsy and Schizophrenia, *The Lancet*, Vol. 18, p. 112 (1996).

247. Boardman, R.H. Epilepsy and schizophrenia, *The Lancet*, Vol. 281, p. 173 (1963).

248. Li, J., Nguyen, L., Gleason, C. *et al.* Lack of evidence for an association between WNT2 and RELN polymorphisms and autism, *American Journal Medical Genetics, B Neuropsychiatric Genetics*, Vol. 126, p. 51–57 (2004).

249. Haas, C.A. Reelin deficiency and displacement of mature neurons, but not neurogenesis, underlie the formation of granule cell dispersion in the epileptic hipocampus, *The Journal of Neuroscience*, Vol. 26, p. 4701–4713 (2006).

250. Westbrook, G.L. Seizures and epilepsy, Chapter 46, p. 927–928, in *Principles of Neural Science*, 4th Ed., Kandel, E.R., Schwartz, J.H. & Jessel, T.M. (Eds.), McGraw-Hill, New York, (1991).

251. Flor-Henry, P. Determinants of psychosis in epilepsy: Laterality and forced normalization, *Biological Psychiatry*, Vol. 18, p. 1045–1057 (1983).

INDEX